Testimonials

"What Should I Eat by Rick Mystrom is a lifesaver for diabetics. It's truly a Diabetes Lifeline."

Richard L. Clinch, RN BSN FCN CHC

"You are about to meet a man who never let diabetes prevent him from accomplishing everything he wanted in life: good health, success in business, community service, family, and politics. Rick Mystrom knew that understanding his disease was crucial to his health. He has become one of the most knowledgeable persons living with diabetes in my extensive practice and frequently serves as a role model and authoritative resource for others."

Jeanne R. Bonar, MD, FACP, FACE
Endocrinology, Internal Medicine

"It is the patient, not the doctor, who manages diabetes. Rick Mystrom is the gold medal winner for controlling his diabetes. He has become so skilled that he can predict and adjust his insulin level just by looking at the meal he is going to eat. His results: no complications from his long history of the disease. He is the expert. I am the learner."

Thomas Nighswander MD MPH

Testimonials continued ...

"I believe the overwhelming message of Rick Mystrom's first book *My Wonderful Life With with Diabetes* is how priceless a positive attitude is in living a great life. Rick's optimism clearly played a dramatic role in his many successes, including how well he has managed a potentially devastating disease. As an ophthalmologist, I have never seen anyone with type 1 diabetes without any evidence of eye damage after a few decades, let alone fifty years after diagnosis! Rick's story is an example for anyone, diabetic or not, to take charge of the challenges in life rather than letting them take charge of you."

Dr. Griff Steiner, MD
Ophthalmology

"If every diabetic, regardless of type, could adopt two of Rick's promises to himself: having a positive attitude and taking personal responsibility for modifying food intake, their improvement in quality of life would be outstanding."

Sue Sampson RN, BSN

"I want you to know, Rick, that your advice and your public discussion of diabetes saved my father's life. Thank you. Thank you. Thank you."

Denise Trutanic
Anchorage, Alaska

Testimonials continued …

"I lost 34 pounds in 9 months after I had just one conversation about eating with Mr. Mystrom. My A1C* went from 10 to 7 in that same time. The funny thing was everybody remarked about how fast I had lost weight. It wasn't fast; it was steady and easy to keep off. He gave me clear, common-sense advice about changing my eating lifestyle. I'm off all my diabetes medications but one and feel so much better now thanks to Mr. Mystrom."

Rabbi Yosef Greenberg
Anchorage, Alaska

A1C is a measure of one's blood sugar for the past 60-90 days. It's a reflection of how well one is managing their diabetes. A lower number is better.

"As parents of a recently diagnosed Type 1 diabetes son, Rick Mystrom's book has not only profoundly impacted his diet but has changed the rest of our family's approach to food. Rick has given us a major contribution that will improve the American diet, leading to a higher quality of life for all. Thank you Rick!"

Bill and Jean Bredar
Anchorage, AK

ISBN 978-1-59433-543-3

eBook ISBN Number: 978-1-59433-544-0

Library of Congress Number: 2015934721

Copyright 2015 Rick Mystrom

—Second Edition—

Manufactured in the United States of America.

Disclaimer

This book is intended as a reference volume only, not as a medical manual. The information contained herein is intended to help you make informed decisions about your health, weight and diabetes management. It is not intended as a substitute for any treatment prescribed by your doctor.

Mention of specific organizations or authorities, or books does not imply endorsement by their authors or publishers.

Table of Contents

Section I

Diabetes—A Sentence to a Shorter Life or An Opportunity for a Longer, Healthier Life

Chapter 1

Chapter 2
The Dangers of High Blood Sugars 41

Chapter 3
The Very Best Medicine for Dealing with
Type 1 or Type 2 Diabetes A Positive Attitude 60

Chapter 4

The Three Elements of a Healthy Diabetes Lifestyle..... 68

Section II

You've Got Diabetes—Or Might Get Diabetes— What Should You Eat?

Chapter 5

How We Get Fat...85

Chapter 6
Visual Impact of Foods on Blood Sugar and Weight..... 111

Sweet Carbohydrates

Starchy Carbohydrates

Fruit Carbohydrates

Fruit Juices

Vegetable Carbohydrates

Protein and Fat

Good Meals, Bad Meals

Yogurt

Blood Glucose and Weight

Chapter 7

Protein, Vegetables, Fat, and Fruit — The Good Guys 177

Chapter 8

The *Diabetes Lifeline Diet*™ 190

Eating at Home

Applying the *Diabetes Lifeline* to Eating

Chapter 9

Getting Started on Your *Diabetes Lifeline Diet*™ 215

Section III

Moderate Changes to Your Activity and Exercise Lifestyle

Chapter 10

Walking and After-Dinner Activity— Your Best Lifelong Activity Lifestyles 223

Chapter 11
A Moderate, Sustainable Exercise Lifestyle "The Type 2 Exercise Program"

Section IV

Better Blood Sugar Control for Type 1 Diabetics and Insulin-Dependent Type 2 Diabetics

Chapter 15

Sports, Activities, and Blood Sugar Control for Insulin-Dependent Diabetics

Preface

I'm a Type 1 diabetic. I was diagnosed at 20 years of age and I'm now 71. I've had diabetes for 51 years and have no health problems. But this book is not just for Type 1 diabetics; it's for Type 2 diabetics, borderline diabetics, prediabetics, and anyone who wants to lose weight and avoid becoming diabetic.

My first book, *My Wonderful Life with Diabetes*, is now out and available nationally. It's the story of how I not only survived Type 1 diabetes for 50 years but how I thrived with it—or maybe because of it.

A few years ago I was playing golf with some friends in Spokane, Washington. I mentioned that I had given myself about 60,000 blood sugar tests and that I knew how hundreds of foods and combinations of foods impacted my blood sugar and weight. They peppered me with questions about healthy and unhealthy foods, what to eat, how to eat, and which foods could help them lose weight and which they should avoid. We talked more about food than anything else and by the time we were ready to leave, they were pushing me to write this book.

This book is different from anything else that's been written about eating right, lowering blood sugar and losing weight. The difference is that this book isn't based on theories; it's based on the 60,000 blood tests I've given myself over the past 30 years. These tests have given me the information I've needed to live a healthy, happy, productive life with Type 1 diabetes for over 50 years. Now I want to share that information with the rest of America.

For me, blood sugar testing was my research. But as often happens in research, when you're looking for one answer, you sometimes find another. I was looking for the impact of food, activity, and exercise on my blood sugar but *what I found was how to live a healthy life*. Now as I approach 70, I'm healthier than most people 20 years younger than I am. In fact I recently took a stress test that showed me equivalent to an "active 42-year-old"—26 years below my chronological age at that time.

For the past two years, I've been conducting and recording structured tests to determine precisely how different foods and different combination of foods impact my blood sugar and therefore my weight. I've graphed these tests and published them in this book. These graphs are based on hundreds of specific blood sugar tests that I gave myself in order to communicate in detail what I have learned in general over the past 35 years while self-testing has been available.

In order to present the most accurate results, I adhered to a consistent protocol in giving myself these tests: stable blood sugars, consistent starting points, always the same time of day, and the same situations.

The purpose of these graphs is to communicate simply and clearly what I have learned from the 60,000 blood tests I have given myself. The graphs provide the core of the information Type 2 diabetics need in order to lower blood sugars, lose weight, and get rid of all symptoms of Type 2 diabetes. They also provide the information that Type 1 diabetics (or parents and loved ones of Type 1 diabetics) need to better control their blood sugars. Even more, the graphs will be instrumental in helping millions of people lose weight and avoid ever getting diabetes in the first place.

Introduction

Few—if any—diseases are as patient-controlled as Type 1 and as patient-solvable as Type 2 diabetes. That's why it's so important for you and your loved ones to understand this disease. If you're a newly diagnosed diabetic, don't view the diagnosis as a sentence to a shorter life but as an opportunity to live a longer, healthier, more enjoyable life.

From the many speeches I've given about diabetes, I've learned that many in my audience don't understand the difference between the two types of diabetes. Knowing the difference is essential to beginning a long healthy life with either Type 1 or Type 2. In Chapter I explain very clearly and simply how the two types differ and how to deal with either type.

Your doctor can diagnose, explain, and get you on the right path but he or she isn't living with diabetes daily like you are. By reading this book and applying what you learn, you'll be on your way to a healthier life from the first day you open it and within months you'll feel better and look better.

What You'll Learn

The understanding I've gained—as a Type 1 diabetic—about health, weight, eating habits, and activity is crucial in helping Type 2 diabetics (whether insulin-dependent or not) lose weight and live healthier—and quite possibly get rid of all the symptoms of diabetes and eliminate the need for insulin shots or oral medications. This book will help prediabetics, borderline diabetics, or any overweight person lose weight and avoid ever becoming diabetic. The information in this book will also help Type 1 diabetics understand how quickly different foods and combinations of foods enter their bloodstream as glucose. This information will contribute greatly to better blood sugar control.

AUTHOR'S NOTE:

I refer to having diabetes for over 50 years, but I refer to about 35 years of learning about foods. The reason for the difference is that for my first 16 years as a diabetic no self-testing was available. In those years, I learned very little about what foods were good for diabetics and what foods weren't. It was the advent of self-testing in the early 1980s that gave me the tool to really understand the impact of foods on blood sugar, health, and weight.

By testing my blood sugar six, eight, or even 10 or more times a day for more than 30 years, I've learned what foods require the least amount of insulin and therefore contribute to weight loss. Conversely I've learned what foods trigger the most insulin demand and therefore are the biggest contributors to weight gain. What has taken me more than 30 years to learn regarding what foods to maximize and what to minimize, you can learn in weeks by reading and understanding this book.

By testing my blood regularly after activities and after exercising, I have also learned what kind of exercises and activities are best, how much you should be doing and when you should do it in order to most effectively control your blood sugar and your weight. You'll also learn why it's important to toss the old, discouraging exercise adage of "no pain, no gain" into the trash can of bad advice.

The Advent of Self-Testing

When self-testing first became accessible just over 30 years ago, I knew that would be the tool to help me truly understand diabetes and live a much healthier life with it. I knew the best way to learn about the impact of diabetes and the impact of food and exercise was constant testing of my blood. I tested every morning when I woke up, I tested before lunch, before exercising, after exercising, before sports competition, sometimes during competition, after competition, before snacks, before dinner, before I went to bed and if I'd wake up in the middle of the night I'd test then. Six, eight, 10 times a day or more I tested. I accepted testing as a part of life and I was committed to it.

I tested so much because I wanted to understand the impact of all different kinds of foods on blood sugar, weight gain, and health. Because *I* tested so much *you* won't necessarily have to test as much. You'll still have to test, of course. It's important to your health and it's a great learning tool. After reading this book and continuing your own blood testing, you'll start to intuitively know the impact most foods will have on your blood sugar and just as important, on your weight.

If you're a Type 1 diabetic you'll be able to look at a meal in front of you and know how much insulin you'll need to take to allow your body to use that meal. If you're a Type 2 diabetic, insulin-dependent or not, you'll know which foods to minimize in order to lower blood sugar and lose weight and which foods you can eat generously with little impact on your weight. If you're a prediabetic or borderline diabetic, you can avoid ever getting diabetes. And if you're one of the more than 200 million overweight Americans, you'll see how you can change that beginning immediately.

For Type 2 diabetics, embracing the advice in this book you will likely eliminate your symptoms of diabetes. Some may call that curing your Type 2 diabetes, others may call it just eliminating the symptoms, but whatever you call it, you will feel better, look better, be slimmer, and be healthier. This book is your jump start to that healthier life.

The *Diabetes Lifeline Diet*™

In this book you'll be introduced to the *Diabetes Lifeline Diet*™. This is not a diet in the conventional sense with a set time to lose weight and then return to your existing eating habits. It's more of an eating lifestyle that will require changing your eating patterns for a few months until those patterns become habits that you do without struggle or thought. Those new habits will be easy for you to maintain and enjoy the rest of your healthier life.

Knowing the impact of the foods you eat on your blood sugar level is so very important for insulin-dependent diabetics, non insulin-dependent diabetics, prediabetics, borderline diabetics, and anyone who wants to lose weight. Eating the wrong foods will raise your blood sugar too fast and too much and result in significant weight gain. Conversely, eating the right foods will reduce blood sugar, reduce insulin demand, and reduce your weight.

Activity and Exercise

Is your eating lifestyle the whole story? No. Activity and exercise also play a role. But what you put into your body is by far and away more important than how you burn it. I'll explain and defend that statement later in this book. But activity and exercise are important and I cover these two friends of good health in Section III.

Don't cringe when I say exercise. This is not a serious bodybuilding regimen, it's a program for people 40 and older or for those who may never have been in a health club. You'll learn how simple changes in your activity and exercise patterns will change your life. These simple, smart lifestyle changes will improve your health, your appearance, your outlook, and your longevity.

By testing my blood so frequently and being so active, I've also learned the impact of all kinds of different activities and sports on blood sugar levels and on weight loss. I've learned about when and how to exercise and when to stop exercising in order to obtain maximum benefit. I've learned how hard is too hard when exercising. I've learned about the huge impact of getting as little as 15 minutes of light exercise—even just walking around the yard, walking to the corner and back, or going shopping—between dinner and going to bed for the night. I've learned the significant value of eating dinner at 5 or 6 p.m. or earlier instead of 7 p.m. or later, and I've learned how to compete in sports and activities without fear of low blood sugar levels.

I've learned a lot about healthy living and this book is about sharing what I've learned with you. It's about the impact that healthy eating, physical activity, and a positive attitude toward diabetes have had on me and can have on you. It's about how Type 2 diabetics and Type 1 diabetics can feel better, look better, and live healthier than they ever dreamed they could. You won't just find theories about which foods are most likely to cause weight increases and which foods are not; you'll see actual tests that show which foods cause quick and significant blood sugar rises and therefore cause weight gain and which foods promote weight loss.

Reading this book is going to be your key to a better life. With the *Diabetes Lifeline Diet™* and simple changes in activity and exercise you will look better, feel better, and live a healthier, longer life. Type 1 diabetics can better control their blood sugars. Type 2 diabetics can eliminate the need for oral medications or insulin. Prediabetics and Borderline Diabetics can avoid ever getting diabetes and all its potential complication.

The bonus for all of these groups (as well as the rest of America) is that you will lose weight.

SECTION

I

Diabetes—A Sentence to a Shorter Life or An Opportunity for a Longer, Healthier Life

For Type 2, Type 1, and Borderline Diabetics or Prediabetics

...And Any Overweight Person who wants to Lose Weight

Chapter 1

Diabetes Simplified

Understanding of Diabetes
from a Patient's Point of View

For all diabetics, prediabetics, borderline diabetics,
and those who want to lose weight and avoid diabetes

Understanding diabetes starts with understanding how the food you eat is converted to energy for your body to use in everyday activities. Most descriptions of diabetes are, of course, written by researchers or doctors, many of whom have in-depth knowledge of the body's chemistry, structural biology, and physiology. In an effort to be as precise as possible, many of their descriptions get too complicated for the typical diabetic, especially a newly diagnosed diabetic. It's my goal to be as clear and understandable as possible as I try to give each of you the understanding you need to deal with Type 1 diabetes, Type 2 diabetes, borderline diabetes, prediabetes, and weight loss.

As a 50-year Type 1 diabetic, I've spent the last 35 years—since self-testing has been available—working to understand the impact of food, activity, and structured exercise on blood sugar and weight. For three years, I structured my research and graphed the results specifically for this book. This testing brings a unique, never-before-done answer to America's commonly asked question. What should I eat?

Throughout this book, the language is simple and straightforward, designed to promote your understanding of diabetes to help you make your own good decisions.

What Happens When a Nondiabetic Eats
or Drinks for Energy and Nourishment

The best way to understand diabetes is to first understand what happens when a *nondiabetic* eats food and converts it to energy. When a nondiabetic eats food, some of that food is converted to glucose. Some foods convert to lots of glucose, other foods to small amounts of glucose. Some foods enter the bloodstream as glucose quickly. Other foods enter the bloodstream as glucose more slowly.

When glucose starts entering the bloodstream it triggers a rise in what is commonly referred to as blood sugar or blood glucose. (In this book I use the two terms interchangeably.) As the blood sugar begins to rise, a signal is sent to the pancreas to start producing insulin, a hormone that allows the glucose that goes into the bloodstream to be absorbed through walls of the bloodstream into the body's cells. In a nondiabetic, the pancreas obliges and produces insulin, which quickly gets into the bloodstream, allowing the glucose (sugar) to get through the walls of the bloodstream into the cells to provide energy to the body. But, very importantly, insulin also allows the excess glucose that isn't used to be stored as fat. That's a very important point to remember. Excess glucose gets stored as fat first in the liver and then around the body in all the places where you don't want it.

When sufficient insulin has been produced to allow the body to use or store the glucose in the bloodstream and the level of glucose in the bloodstream drops back down to normal levels, the pancreas stops sending any more insulin to the bloodstream and the blood sugar stabilizes at that normal* level.

Think of it this way. It's like heating a house in the winter using a thermostat. When the house gets too cold, the thermostat sends a message to the furnace that says, "Turn on the heat." When the furnace brings the heat up to the set (normal) temperature, the thermostat sends the signal to stop sending up heat.

That's the way things are supposed to work. But what if the pancreas doesn't produce any insulin or doesn't produce enough insulin? That's the challenge Type 1 or Type 2 diabetics have and borderline, or prediabetics, will have if they don't take preventative action.

AUTHOR'S NOTE:

Normal level is generally considered to be between 75 and 105 mg/dl (that's milligrams of sugar (glucose) per deciliter of blood). You don't need to remember the "milligrams per deciliter" part but you do need to know the term, blood sugar *and what the normal, healthy level is.*

What Happens When a Type 1 diabetic Eats or Drinks for Energy and Nourishment

Now we know what happens when a nondiabetic eats (or drinks), but what happens when an *untreated* Type 1 diabetic eats food? Well it's the same as for a nondiabetic—up to a point.

When a Type 1 diabetic eats food, some of that food is converted to glucose and absorbed through the stomach lining and into the bloodstream just as it is with a nondiabetic. When the glucose starts entering the bloodstream it triggers a rise in blood sugar just as it does in a nondiabetic. As the blood sugar begins to rise, the pancreas gets a signal to start producing insulin so the body can use or store the energy the blood sugar will provide.

This is where things change. The pancreas says, "Sorry, I don't do that anymore."

With no insulin being produced, the glucose can't get out of the bloodstream into the cells to provide energy to the body. Consequently, if no insulin is injected, the blood sugar just gets higher and higher until eventually it reaches a level—called the renal threshold—high enough to spill into the kidneys and ultimately out the urethra as sugar in the urine. Thus, sugar in the urine is an early symptom of diabetes. High blood sugars also trigger more frequent urination as the kidneys try to rid themselves of the excess sugar. A noticeable increase in the frequency of urination is often the first and most commonly noticed symptom of the onset of Type 1 diabetes.

Since the Type 1 diabetic in this example is not yet injecting insulin, the sugar continues to collect in the bloodstream but cannot get through the bloodstream walls to the body's cells, which need the energy and nourishment. The body's cells are screaming for nutrients so they can function. If the cells can't get the nourishment they now desperately need, the body starts burning its own fat. That doesn't work very well because fat molecules are stable and hard to break down to function as energy supplies. In this process, they are often only partially broken down and the unused portions of the fat molecules are called ketones or acetones. When the ketones or acetones start showing up in the urine it indicates keto-acidosis, another result of untreated or poorly treated Type 1 diabetes. The undiagnosed Type 1 diabetic then starts feeling lethargic, weak, and flulike.

Prior to the discovery of insulin, the life expectancy of Type 1 diabetics was short indeed. Typically, they lived for just months after diagnosis and during that time they were so weak and so sick that they couldn't perform routine life activities. The discovery of insulin in the early 1920s by Dr. Frederick Banting and Charles Best, working at the University of Toronto, changed the life expectancy for Type 1 diabetics from just months to multiple decades and changed the quality and functionality of life dramatically.

It was in January, 1922 in Toronto, Canada that a 14-year-old boy, Leonard Thompson, was chosen as the first person with diabetes to receive insulin. The test was a dramatic success. Leonard, who before the insulin shots was near death, rapidly regained his strength and appetite. The team then expanded their testing to other volunteer diabetics, who reacted just as positively as Leonard to the insulin extract.

Magic stuff, that insulin. But one shot obviously doesn't solve the problem forever. A daily regimen of insulin injection or infusion will be required for Type 1 diabetics, hence the term *insulin-dependent*. As research continues and technology improves, this requirement for daily injections or infusions from an insulin pump may change. But for now, your best path is to understand diabetes treatment as it is today. At this stage of medical advancement, most Type 1 diabetics will require outside insulin infusions or injections for the rest of their lives.

The rest of one's life always sounds intimidating, but with the right attitude it can become a part of your life that will teach you so much about food that with a positive attitude and a good understanding of diabetes, you can live healthier and longer than most of your peers. Because I've learned so much about food and health, I often tell people that I believe I'm healthier now than I would have been if I hadn't contracted Type 1 diabetes 50 years ago. It can be hard at first but this book will help your journey with diabetes be a good one.

What Happens When a Type 2 Diabetic Eats *or Drinks* for Energy and Nourishment?

The process for a Type 2 diabetic before diagnosis and corrective action is also the same as for a nondiabetic—up to a point.

When an untreated Type 2 diabetic eats food, some of that food is absorbed through the stomach walls and enters into the bloodstream as glucose just as it does with a nondiabetic and a Type 1 diabetic. When the glucose starts entering the bloodstream it triggers a rise in blood sugar. As the blood sugar begins to rise, the pancreas gets a signal to start producing insulin.

This is where things change. In a Type 2 diabetic the pancreas says, "I've been working too hard trying to produce the insulin needed for all the glucose you've been creating. I'm worn out and I can't produce all the insulin you need. But I will produce what I can and hope it helps." Implicit in this message is that if the Type 2 diabetic will reduce the amount of glucose in the bloodstream, it will reduce the demand for insulin and the pancreas will likely be able to produce sufficient insulin to meet that demand.

This is essentially the difference between Type 1 and Type 2 diabetes. In a Type 1 diabetic, no insulin is produced. In a Type 2 diabetic the pancreas is producing some insulin but not enough to get *all* the glucose out of the bloodstream and into the cells that need the glucose for energy, nourishment, and storage.

This insufficiency of insulin may be related to weight, heredity, ethnicity, poor diet, sedentary life style, or age. Most likely it's some combination of these characteristics, but getting older and heavier is the most common journey to Type 2 diabetes. We can't do much about getting older; in fact, that's better than the alternative. But we can do something about getting heavier and that's the focus of this book.

Characteristics of Type 2 Diabetes Compared to Type 1 Diabetes

Type 2 diabetes is much slower to develop than Type 1 and is therefore much more subtle. It may be present for years before it is discovered.

Type 2 diabetics can sometimes be treated with oral medications that will stimulate the pancreas to produce more insulin or make the insulin it's producing more effective. However, some Type 2 diabetics need insulin injections to supplement the insulin their bodies are producing. Whether a Type 2 diabetic is taking oral medications or injecting insulin, he or she will typically not have the big swings in blood sugar a Type 1 will have, because the partially working pancreas is a moderating force.

The best news of all for a Type 2 diabetic is that many, if not most, can eliminate all the symptoms of diabetes and rid themselves of the need to take any medication by changing their lifestyle. Some may call that a cure of diabetes and some may say that's just eliminating the symptoms. Whichever is correct, the end result is that your body will act just like a healthy nondiabetic's, and that's very good news.

Type 2 diabetes is usually contracted later in life than Type 1 diabetes. Type 1 diabetics are typically—but not always— diagnosed between birth and their late 20s and the onset is not related to lifestyle habits or weight. Type 2 diabetics are commonly diagnosed from their 40s on, and the onset is very often— but again not always— related to a less-than-healthy lifestyle. This combination of factors means that Type 2 diabetics have a shorter period of time than Type 1 diabetics to accept the diagnosis and create the new lifestyle necessary for a long, healthy life.

Are Type 2 Diabetics Who Use Insulin Really "Insulin-Dependent" or Are They Just "Insulin-Assisted"?

In the early stages of medical distinction between the two types of diabetes, I wish the term used to describe Type 2 diabetics who use insulin had been established as *insulin-assisted*, not *insulin-dependent*. As a Type 2 diabetic, you may need that insulin assistance now but many of you, if you can make some key changes in your eating lifestyle, won't need that assistance from either insulin or oral medication in the future. This book will show you what changes you need to make and how to make those changes.

Desert Island Parable

Here's a story I use periodically in my speeches. The more you learn about diabetes, the more you'll understand this short parable.

A Type 1 diabetic and a Type 2 diabetic are marooned on a desert island. Neither has any insulin; however, they do have a way to make fires and the island does have catchable fish, edible plants, and drinkable water.

Despite access to the nourishment needed to survive, but with no insulin, the Type 1 diabetic would likely be dead in months. In about that same period of time, the Type 2 diabetic would be cured.

Think about this parable as you continue reading this book.

When you're finished, return and read this again. You'll completely understand.

Prediabetics, Borderline Diabetics, and All Overweight People

In addition to Type 1 and Type 2 diabetics, the third group of people who will benefit greatly from the information in this book are those folks who are overweight. Even though you may have no symptoms of diabetes, you are much more likely to get diabetes than those who are not overweight. Although a number of issues—including heredity and ethnicity—influence the likelihood of someone getting Type 2 diabetes, no one characteristic is more closely related to Type 2 diabetes than excessive weight.

The most common estimate in the books I've read regarding diabetes is that about 80 percent of Type 2 diabetics are overweight or obese. When you combine that statistic with the Center for Disease Control's estimate that about one third of Americans are obese and another one third are just overweight, you can understand the huge increases in Type 2 diabetes. (See graph on following page). As you review the dramatic increases in Diabetes in the USA as shown in this graph, make note of the fact that 1980 was the adoption of the Food Pyramid recommended by a US Senate Sub-committee chaired by Senator George McGovern. That year represented the beginning of the obesity and Type 2 diabetic epidemic in the United States. A more recent report from the *National Diabetes Statistics Report,* 2014 indicate the number of diabetics in the United States as closer to 30 million. Other estimates number prediabetics and borderline diabetics as high as 50 million.

NUMBER *(in Millions)* OF CIVILIAN, NONINSTITUTIONALIZED PERSONS WITH DIAGNOSED DIABETES, UNITED STATES, 1980–2011

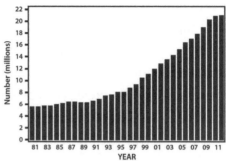

Diabetes is becoming more common in the United States. From 1980 through 2011, the number of Americans with diagnosed diabetes has more than tripled (from 5.6 million to 20.9 million).

DATA SOURCE: Centers for Disease Control and Prevention, National Center for Health Statistics, Division of Health Interview Statistics, data from the National Health Interview Survey. Statistical analysis by the Centers for Disease Control and Prevention, National Center for Chronic Disease Prevention and Health Promotion, Division of Diabetes Translation.

If you're overweight or obese, the information in this book regarding a healthy eating lifestyle applies directly to you too. Even though your blood sugar will not go up like a diabetic's would when you eat the wrong foods, the impact on your weight will be as significant as the weight gain for a diabetic. The difference is that your pancreas is currently producing all the insulin you need to provide energy and store fat from the food you eat. So the foods I identify as causing weight gain *and* blood sugar rises for diabetics will cause only weight gain for nondiabetics. The rise in blood sugar will not manifest itself.

As you look at the graphs in chapter 6 showing the impact of different foods and combinations of foods on blood sugar and weight gain, Type 2 diabetics, borderline diabetics, and prediabetics should pay close attention to the peak of the graphs and the size of the gray shaded area in each graph. The peak represents the rise in blood sugar that a Type 2 diabetic's pancreas is trying to lower, and the shaded area is a general representation of that food's or combination of foods' contribution to the weight of diabetics and nondiabetics alike.

To assure your long-term good health as a diabetic, to lose weight, and/or to avoid getting Type 2 diabetes, you need to have an understanding of the disease, a desire to be healthy, a positive attitude, and knowledge of what foods you should be eating. Subsequent chapters will give you an understanding of foods that will be life-changing. But before we get to that information, I need to provide a little more motivation for you to make healthy changes. This next chapter will highlight some problems you could face if you don't keep your blood sugar and weight under control.

Chapter 2

The Dangers of High Blood Sugars

Your Blood Sugar's High but You Feel Fine. What's the Problem?

Ignoring High Blood Sugars

Over and over I hear the same quiet and melancholy reflections from middle-aged and older Type 1 and Type 2 diabetics who may be suffering from circulatory problems, kidney failure, serious vision problems, foot sores, or foot ulcers—"I should have taken my high blood sugars more seriously," or "I wish I had been more conscientious about my blood sugars years ago." It's sad to hear those comments but in some ways they are very understandable.

Why don't high blood sugars get the attention of so many diabetics? Based on my experience, the biggest reason diabetics often let blood sugar levels drift high—and remain higher than appropriate—is the lack of immediate negative feedback from their bodies. If your blood sugar gets too *low*, you know it. I mean right away. You're in danger and you better do something—right now. But high blood sugars are more subtle than low blood sugars and can be harder to identify until they reach a very high and very unhealthy point. With normal considered in the 75-to-105 mg/dl range, what happens when your blood sugar gets up to 120? What do you feel?—*Nothing*. How about 140? Still *nothing*. What about 160? 180? You still feel normal. How can you be sick if you feel normal?

Maybe at 200 mg/dl or higher you might feel just a little off. You can't put your finger on it but you don't feel great. By the time your blood sugar gets to 300, you usually can feel it. It feels like you might be getting the flu. You're not really sick but you feel just a little under the weather. Even then, you're in no *immediate* danger so you'll have a tendency to not treat it as seriously as you should.

My sensitivity to high blood sugars has changed a little as I've grown older. When I was in my 20s and 30s, before blood sugar self-testing became available, I didn't feel high blood sugars until, I think, I was in the 300s or low 400s. I don't know for sure because the only way I could find out was if a doctor ordered a lab test for me. By the time I reached my 60s I could feel high blood sugars in the mid-200 range.

Because there were no mechanisms for self-measurement in my younger, more transient years other than the very inefficient urine tests, I knew what my blood sugar was only two or three times a year when I visited a doctor in whatever town I happened to be living. Now I believe, based on thousands of blood tests since then, my blood sugars were probably pretty high much of the time. Somehow, healthy eating habits, a very active lifestyle, a lot of competitive sports, and some pretty lucky estimating got me by until self-testing became available.

The Long-Term Consequences of High Blood Sugars

As a key part of your background, you need to understand what is likely to happen if you are careless or indifferent in your blood sugar control. And you need to know why so many diabetics regret their inattention or indifference to high blood sugars years later. This is going to be a pretty scary chapter to read but remember that all the serious consequences I talk about can be avoided. If you're already experiencing some of these problems, their progression can be slowed, and many can even be reversed.

So look at this section not as *what will happen to you* but rather as *what can be avoided by you* by applying what you learn in this book.

When I talk about the consequences of long-term high blood sugar, what do I mean? *Long-term* is totally dependent on the age and physical condition of a diabetic when he or she is diagnosed. For example, it stands to reason that a newly diagnosed young diabetic is starting his or her life as a diabetic with a healthier circulatory system, healthier kidneys, and a healthier heart than a newly diagnosed 60-year-old Type 2 diabetic.

What that means is that the young person has more time to learn about dealing with diabetes and to develop the habits he or she needs in order to live a long and healthy life. Certainly it's better for the young person to learn quickly but, as in my case, a slower adaptation is likely going to be less damaging to a younger diabetic than to an older diabetic.

The older Type 2 diabetic, whether insulin-dependent or not, does not have the luxury of taking a lot of time to change habits. Five or 10 years of high blood sugars for a 40-, 50-, 60-, or 70-year-old can have a very negative impact on health and survivability whereas five or 10 years of higher-than-ideal blood sugars for a younger person will not have as significant an impact.

This is a big problem that must be taken seriously by people diagnosed with diabetes later in life. If you're diagnosed with Type 2 diabetes (insulin-dependent or not) you don't have the luxury of five or 10 years before you need to start changing your habits. You need to begin acting now. In future chapters I spend a lot of time talking about eating patterns and habits and activity or exercise patterns and habits. You will be amazed and pleased at both the immediate and lifelong impact of changing your food choices. And when that change is combined with a moderate but consistent exercise pattern and a slightly more active lifestyle, you're on your way to a healthier life immediately.

The Problems You Want to Avoid

Although there is no *immediate* danger in periodic high blood sugars, there certainly are very severe long-term consequences to frequent and continual high blood sugars over an extended period of time. High blood sugars over an extended period of time can contribute directly to circulatory problems—which in the long term may lead to heart problems, vision impairment, and even blindness. They also contribute to kidney failure and loss of feeling in your feet (neuropathy). This loss of feeling in your feet means you won't feel punctures, lacerations, abrasions, or blisters in your feet, which untreated or unhealed can lead to amputation of toes, feet, or even legs.

Whew. I'm glad that paragraph's done. Okay, now you know generally why you need to work at normalizing your blood sugars. Now let's get into some specifics so you understand why high blood sugar causes these problems and why it's so important you work to prevent these problems from occurring.

The very comprehensive 9-year Diabetic Control and Complications Trial (Often referred to as the DCCT study) established conclusively that *for all diabetics the better their control the less likely they are to have complications and the worse their control, the more likely they are to have complications.* These complications are universally referred to as "diabetic complications" and should be a part of your regular discussions with your doctor. Because nearly every book written by doctors or medical professionals about diabetes goes into some level of detail about the diabetic complications, I won't attempt, nor am I qualified, to explain the chemistry or biology behind them. The description of the complications and some of my personal experiences will hopefully serve as a reminder of the seriousness of diabetes and as a motivator to apply what you learn in this book to your own life in order to avoid these issues.

1. Vision Impairment and Blindness

The diabetic vision issues generally referred to as *retinopathy* are caused by clogging of the tiny blood capillaries in the eye. These micro-vessels get partially blocked and form what are called aneurisms. *Aneurisms* are bulges in those tiny capillaries that may sometimes burst. If they do burst and if the blood blocks the macula portion of the eye, vision is instantly impaired. In most cases burst aneurisms can be treated by laser. In the early '80s, when I was 36, my doctor, Jeanne Bonar, wanted me to start biannual visits to an ophthalmologist. She explained that this was important in tracking the success or lack of success of my diabetic control. You should ask your doctor whether or not you should be seeing an ophthalmologist.

The tiny capillaries in the retina are the only blood vessels in the body that are externally visible. These capillaries are a window to your diabetic health. Problems with those capillaries indicate that you need to improve your control. Problem-free capillaries indicate that you're doing well with your control.

My first visit to Dr. Swanson, an ophthalmologist in Anchorage, was in late 1981 or early 1982, about the time I got my pump. He discovered what he called background retinopathy. He explained that I had some small aneurisms in both eyes. They were quite minor and not an immediate worry. But if they got worse, the capillaries could burst and cause blockage of the macula, which could impair my vision.

That first visit and subsequent biannual visits certainly added to my commitment to improve my control. Fortunately, about that time I started using a pump and a glucose monitor, both of which dramatically improved my control, the health of my eyes, and the health of my life. For the past 10 years, my current ophthalmologist, Dr. Griff Steiner, has monitored my eyes. During a biannual eye exam in 2011, he told me the aneurisms had gradually disappeared in one eye and diminished to the point of near disappearance in the other eye. When he finished his exam, he stood up, smiled and said, "I can hardly tell you have diabetes." That was one of those simple, straightforward statements that I'll never forget, especially after having had diabetes for over 47 years at that time. Even better, during my last visit in 2013, Dr. Steiner told me that my aneurisms had completely disappeared in both eyes. The lesson here is some diabetic complications can be reversed.

I'm convinced that regular visits to an ophthalmologist will open a clear and helpful window into your health as a diabetic and whether your visits result in a positive report or not, I believe that when you leave the office you'll be inspired to keep working on good or better blood sugar control.

2. Foot Problems: Neuropathy and Angiopathy

Neuropathy, as I mentioned earlier, is a loss of feeling in the extremities, most often in the feet. The danger here is with the potential for blisters and small injuries to the feet to go unnoticed and become serious problems before they are addressed. A common complication of poorly controlled diabetes is impaired circulation, which often manifests itself in the feet first. So injuries or blisters that may occur in your feet while you can't feel their onset are complicated by the fact that poor long-term diabetic care also results in limited circulation in your feet, which makes healing much more difficult and injuries to your feet much more serious. This is a more significant problem for longer-term, older diabetics than it is for younger diabetics, since circulation is naturally diminished as a function of age. These foot problems are typically exacerbated by the length of time a person has poorly controlled diabetes.

It's very important for older or longer-term diabetics to establish a relationship with a podiatrist. I've done that and have learned a lot about foot problems and care from Dr. Ken Swayman, an Anchorage podiatrist. Dr. Swayman is an excellent communicator, who has helped me immensely with a toe problem that provides a perfect illustration of what can happen when diabetes-caused neuropathy comes into play.

The only complication I have so far from diabetes after nearly 50 years is a moderate loss of feeling in my feet (neuropathy). This neuropathy has caused me a few problems in the past dozen or so years. To avoid blisters—which I may not feel—I use well-broken-in, comfortable golf shoes and tend to stick with the brand of tennis or athletic shoes that have proven to be friends of my feet.

Until the summer of 2011, I hadn't had a diabetic-related foot problem. That summer I spent quite a bit of time barefoot around our lake (being barefoot is a bad idea for long-term diabetics). I didn't know I had a problem until I went to get a pedicure—the second one of my life. As the pedicurist was working on my right foot, she looked up at me and said, "Rick, you've got a hole in your big toe." It turned out to be pretty deep and looked like it was quite a few weeks old.

Since we had a family reunion coming up, I pretty much ignored the toe issue and continued being active with my extended family for the full week of the reunion. Soon after the reunion ended I went to see Dr. Bonar. She was concerned and told me because the sore was so deep it could take a long time to heal. She then said, "If you stay off your feet for a few weeks it will heal much faster." Well, the chances of my staying off my feet for a few weeks in midsummer in Alaska were pretty slim.

After about six weeks and some slow big-toe healing progress— because I hadn't stayed off my feet—two of my golfing buddies, Dave Young and Rick Pollock, called me for a round of golf. At first I didn't think I should do it but then came up with what I thought was a great idea. I'd use my jigsaw and cut a notch in my golf sandals under my big toe, effectively taking all the pressure off that toe and not aggravating the injury. "Great idea," I thought. But not only did I get solidly beaten by Rick, who shot his best game of the year, but when I returned to my car and took off my sandals, the bottom of my white sock was covered with blood. It was a total surprise. My big toe had no pressure on it and was in effect suspended above the ground as I walked. How could that be injured?

What happened was a good lesson for me and for others who may be pushing themselves and not allowing proper healing time. By taking all the pressure off my big toe, I put far more pressure on my second toe than it had ever had, resulting in a serious-looking bloody blister on that toe. Because of my lack of feeling in my feet I hadn't felt the blister developing. I had protected my big toe at the expense of my second toe.

With the help of Dr. Swayman, the big toe injury healed a few weeks later but the second toe injury was very slow to heal.

Why did I spend so much time telling you about this seemingly insignificant injury? It's very simple and very important. Not only are foot problems the most frequent cause of hospitalization among diabetics, but also, diabetes is the biggest cause of amputations in the United States. Over 100,000 diabetes-related amputations of toes, feet, or legs were performed last year alone and many started with toe lacerations, abrasions, or blisters.

I have to confess that when I didn't see much progress in the healing of my second toe, the thought of having it amputated passed briefly through my mind. I reasoned it surely wouldn't be as big a deal as having my big toe amputated. I happened to mention that passing thought to a friend of mine who practices orthotics and prosthetics. She discouraged that idea quickly and definitively by saying, "That's not a solution. That's just the beginning of future problems." I was glad for that advice since everything is now completely healed.

As a result of that experience, I'm now much more careful and much more observant of my feet. I put Cetaphil moisturizing cream on them every morning and keep a hand mirror in my nightstand so I can check my feet for injuries that I may not feel. But an even better solution is to maintain good blood sugar control and not give sensory or circulatory problems a foothold.

If you're a middle-aged or older diabetic, your feet deserve attention. If your control is not good, your feet may very well be the first indicator that you need to improve your blood sugar control. You should be asking your doctor if he or she thinks you should start seeing a podiatrist. You'll learn a lot and likely postpone or completely avoid some serious problems. Just because you may have neuropathy, it's not necessarily a precursor to amputation. Most long-term or older diabetics will develop some neuropathy but only a small minority will require amputation. That's a minority you don't want to be a part of.

This is such an important issue I've provided here information from Dr. Swayman and the Alaska Podiatry Associates.

Three major causes of foot problems in diabetes

Nerve damage (neuropathy)
This causes loss of feeling in the foot, which normally protects the foot from injury. The protective sensations of sharp/dull, hot /cold pressure and vibration become altered or lost completely. Furthermore, nerve damage causes toe deformities, collapse of the arch, and dry skin. These problems may result in foot ulcers and infections, which may progress rapidly to gangrene and amputation. However: Daily foot care and regular visits to the podiatrist can prevent ulcerations and infections.

Loss of circulation (angiopathy)
Poor circulation may be difficult to treat. If circulation is poor, gangrene and amputation may be unavoidable. Cigarette smoking should be avoided. Smoking can significantly reduce the circulation to the feet. Certain medications are available for improving circulation and by-pass surgery may be necessary to improve circulation to the feet. Chelation therapy is an alternative form of treatment for circulatory problems that is not well recognized by the medical community at large. Daily foot care and regular visits to the podiatrist can often prevent or delay the need for amputation.

Changes in the shape of your foot

Changes in the shape of your foot or toes can be caused or accelerated by diabetes. These changes can lead to blisters and foot ulcers. If you notice any change in bone structure or foot shape you should contact your doctor or a podiatrist promptly.

Taking Care of Your Feet If You Have Diabetes

The following is recommended by the Alaska Podiatry Associates, also referred to as The Alliance Foot and Ankle Center.

The very first action recommended by the Alliance Foot and Ankle center in Anchorage for diabetics to prevent or delay diabetes-related foot problems is to take care of your diabetes. Specifically, here are some of their recommendations:

➡ Make healthy lifestyle choices to help keep your blood glucose (sugar),blood pressure, and cholesterol close to normal. Doing so may help prevent or delay diabetes-related foot problems as well as eye and kidney disease.

➡ Know when to test your A1C*, blood pressure, and cholesterol.

➡ Know how and when to test your blood glucose (sugar).

➡ Eat regular meals that contain a variety of healthy, low-fat*, high-fiber foods including fruits and vegetables each day."

➡ Get physical activity each day.

AUTHOR'S NOTE:

As you'll learn later in this book, I don't agree with low-fat foods being an essential part of a healthy eating pattern for diabetics. Fat is very slow to metabolize and, as you will see in future chapters, has a very stabilizing impact on blood sugar. I do agree with all the other recommendations by the Alliance Foot and Ankle Center of the Alaska Podiatry Associates, Anchorage, Alaska.

⯈ Stop smoking.

⯈ Follow your foot care plan.

⯈ Have your feet, eyes, and kidneys checked at
least once a year.

Keeping your feet healthy and avoiding or delaying foot problems is just one more payoff of keeping your diabetes in good control.

3. Kidney Disease

Kidney disease is another potential problem with diabetes that can be avoided with good blood sugar control. Fortunately, I don't have any personal experience with kidney disease but I do have a basic understanding of the kidney function and do have friends who are dealing with kidney issues.

In everyday language, the role of kidneys is to filter waste products out of the bloodstream and into the urine for elimination from the body. When the kidneys stop working properly, some products from the blood, such as protein, start showing up in the urine. This is usually the first indication of kidney problems. At this early stage there are typically no other noticeable symptoms. The kidneys are also responsible for maintaining a balance between water and salt in your bloodstream. When the kidneys are not functioning properly an imbalance can occur which will often create a significant rise in blood pressure.

Like other diabetic complications, this has a direct relationship to blood sugar. My friend and golfing buddy, Dr. Rob Bennedetti, a nephrologist at the Rockwood Clinic in Spokane, says the most common causes of kidney problems are high blood sugar, high blood pressure, and excessive doses of over-the-counter pain medication. The more normal or controlled the blood sugar and blood pressure, the less likely that any kidney problems will occur. The more consistently high the blood sugar, the more likely they will occur. You should ask your doctor about periodic urine tests to determine if any early indication of kidney disease is present. An excellent and more detailed explanation of diabetic kidney disease is contained in *The Johns Hopkins Guide to Diabetes* by Christopher D. Saudek, M.D., Richard R. Rubin, Ph.D., and Cynthia S. Shump, R.N., pages 310-313.

4. Arteriosclerosis

The heart, the brain, the eyes, and the legs can all be affected by arteriosclerosis. It can be caused by a number of factors, only one of which is diabetes. Family history, high cholesterol ratios, high triglycerides, smoking, high blood pressure, lack of exercise or activity, poorly controlled diabetes, and aging in general are all factors that contribute to heart disease.

Because diabetes is only one of a number of contributing factors, I won't spend much time on this except to share my version of a healthy heart scorecard. I suggest that you **grade yourself** on each of these six factors. Use the standard grading system of A=4 points, B=3 points, C=2, D=1 and F=0. Here's how I assess my heart health. After you read this, do the same for yourself.

First, my **family history** is mixed. My dad died of his second heart attack at age 54 but my mom lived to be 94. My grandfather on my mom's side lived to be 95 and my great-grandmother on my mom's side, Grandma Deen (short for her last name, Lundeen), who was born in Sweden and lived in Chisago City, Minnesota, was just two months short of 106 years old when she died. She spoke only Swedish and I spoke only English, but we talked to each other, each in our own language, smiled and hugged. I was 13 when she died and she was 13 when Lincoln gave his Gettysburg Address. Every bit as impressive was my great-grandfather on my father's side, Gustav Myrstrom (somewhere along the line the *r* got dropped) who fathered his last child at age 72. Now that's a bit of history and, I hope, heredity that I'm very happy about. Way to go, Gustav.

My grade on "family heredity": **B-**. It's mixed but probably better than average.

My **cholesterol and triglycerides** test well. My ratio of total cholesterol to HDL and LDL to HDL continues to be very healthy. I know my family is surprised at that because I do eat a lot of butter which leads to increases weight, cholesterol and triglycerides and is bad for your heart. Right? Hold on here. It's certainly not true for me and more and more science is saying it's not true for anyone.

Over the past 30 plus years since self-testing became available, I've gradually increased the amount of butter I've eaten. Two reasons I've increased my butter consumption: first, it improves the taste of so many foods and second, it never seemed to raise my blood sugar much.

In the back of my mind I still couldn't quite reconcile the fact that butter—while not contributing to higher blood sugar or to my weight, or to any evidence of arteriosclerosis—could be healthy on a larger picture.

On June 23, 2014, *Time Magazine's* cover headlined the words **Eat Butter**. The sub-head declared **Scientists labeled fat the enemy. Why they were wrong.**

Runner's World Magazine for January/February, 2015 in a story titled *Eat Fat, Be Fit* led the story as follows:

> "Runners like to follow the rules. And for decades, nutrition rules put a strict limit on saturated fat. After all, as far back as the 1960s, experts have decreed that eating foods high in saturated fat such as eggs, red meat, and full-fat dairy, will increase your risk of heart disease. So runners took heed, all but banishing those foods from their diets.

But a string of news-making studies has flipped that idea on its head. One of those headline-catchers published in the Annals of Internal Medicine early last year, reviewed 76 existing studies and found no association between saturated fat and heart disease....The new emerging thought: 'Saturated fat may not be the demon that it was made out to be,' says Jeff Volek, Ph.D., R.D., associate professor in the department of kinesiology at the University of Connecticut."

I've become more aligned in my thinking with the growing number of researchers and doctors who no longer believe fat is the villain it has been made out to be.

In the words of Dr. John Mues, an internal medicine specialist, a friend of mine, and a well-conditioned 60-year-old athlete, "Fat is your friend" (much more on this in Section 2).

My grade on "cholesterol and triglycerides": **A**. My eating habits and activity level are very good and that reflects in my blood profile.

Smoking is a habit I've never succumbed to though on golf trips my good friend, Curt Nading, often brings a selection of good cigars for the whole group of golfers. I do enjoy a cigar with a drink or two after golf and dinner but lately Curt quit offering them to me. I think it's because I periodically offered to pay him back with Swisher Sweets, a much cheaper cigar that is marketed to folks who are somewhere between penurious and stingy.

My grade on smoking: **A**. Thanks, Curt for cutting me off.

My **blood pressure** has been rock-solid all my life. It rarely varies more than a few points from 120 over 70.

My grade on blood pressure: **A+**. I credit an active lifestyle and good eating habits.

The next factor is **diabetes control**. As I said earlier, my first 16 years as a diabetic, prior to self-testing, were probably not well-controlled. The last 34 years have been pretty darn good.

My overall diabetes control: **A-**. I give more weight to the last 34 years.

The next factor is **exercise or activity**. This is where I've done well: moving, playing, competing, exercising, and just doing a lot of stuff.

Without even thinking about it, I've done my circulatory system and heart a big favor.

My grade on activity and exercise: **A+**. It's been fun.

The last factor is **age.** This will certainly bring my heart health score down. The late 60s and early 70s are a time in one's life that the health of the heart should always be considered with care and concern. Be vigilant about it.

My age grade: **C-**. My heart may be healthy but it's still 70 years old.

So here's my tally: Five A's, one B and one C: that's 25 points total divided by 7 equals a 3.5 average or a grade of **B+**.

This is simply an exercise to help you decide if your heart health needs to be front and center on your radar screen or not. If you ended up with a C or D you should give your heart health the attention it deserves and talk to your doctor about it.

Avoiding These Deadly Complications

As you read these complications as a package, they can be very scary. But remember this: *These complications are all avoidable.* If you already have one or more of these complications, the negative impact of the complication(s) can in most cases be dramatically slowed and in some cases reversed by making changes based on recommendations in this book, by being smart about using the tools available, and by applying the knowledge you'll have by the time you finish this book.

Glucose Testers and Insulin Pumps

In my opinion, the most valuable tool for diabetes control is the **glucose-testing meter**. The availability of these meters and the ease and quickness of being able to test blood sugars is, in my opinion, the biggest advancement in helping diabetics achieve long-term health since the discovery and development of insulin in the 1920s. Blood sugar testing meters are critical for all diabetics, insulin-dependent or not. They will help insulin-dependent diabetics learn how to balance the three factors that control blood sugar: food, insulin, and exercise. By testing you will also learn over time what foods cause the greatest rise in your blood sugar. For non-insulin-dependent diabetics, understanding what foods cause the greatest rise in blood sugar is critical. By minimizing these foods and shifting more to foods that do not cause large rises in blood sugars, you can better control your blood sugar and reduce your weight. Chapters 5 to 9 will provide a great foundation for healthy eating and excellent blood sugar control.

Right behind the blood-testing meter as a tool for improving the health of diabetics are the incredibly reliable **insulin pumps**. I've used a Medtonic pump for the last two decades and am very satisfied with their product. These, of course, are only for insulin-dependent diabetics. Although I don't consider pumps absolutely essential for long-term health, they are in my opinion highly desirable. They provide great flexibility in what and when you eat. They allow you to respond quickly to normalize high blood sugars, and are very helpful in maintaining normal blood sugars when you are sleeping. Overall, the pump has worked wonderfully for me and I will cover my experiences with my pumps in much more detail in section IV.

High Blood Sugars at an Early Age

The challenge for parents of young diabetics is what level of perfection in blood sugar levels you want to strive for without creating too much anxiety and fear of abnormality in your child. My experience with high blood sugars at an early age may give comfort and guidance to young diabetics and parents of young diabetics.

By the early 1980s, when I began self-testing regularly, I began to realize that some of the things I had done in the days before self-testing had helped keep my blood sugars probably high much of the time. Like most diabetics in the '60s and early '70s, I felt that the best way to avoid the dangers of low blood sugar was to err on the high side. Because we now have the technology to test as many times as needed or desired, there is no need to always err on the high side for safety.

Before the advent of self-testing, I almost always ate a candy bar before any competition. That was actually a good idea then because it freed me from the distraction of worrying about a low blood sugar episode during that competition.

Since in those days I was using long-lasting insulin, I knew that I had insulin going into my body throughout the night, so to avoid having a nighttime low blood sugar, I'd eat some kind of carbohydrate or sweet before I went to bed. That was generally a bad idea. But during those early years, it was my defense against nighttime low blood sugars.

Back then I typically ate a breakfast of cereal, toast, and a big glass of orange juice. After testing became available, I quickly learned that kind of a breakfast will skyrocket blood sugars and contribute significantly to weight gain as you will see in later chapters.

When I was in my 20s, I probably went to a doctor only once or twice a year. When I did go and when a blood sample was taken the process was cumbersome and unrevealing. I typically didn't get results for three or more days. My blood sugar was often in the 200–300mg/dl range.

Although my blood sugar was often high during my 20s and early 30s, I was very active. I played on sports teams year round and generally had good eating habits. Now I'm approaching 70 and healthier than most people 10 or 20 years younger than I am. After nearly 50 years as a diabetic, I have no evidence of kidney problems, no vision problems, no circulatory impairment, and no blood pressure problems, and I'm still very active in sports year around. In a lot of ways, I think my active lifestyle compensated for my "too high" blood sugars in my early years with diabetes.

This is not meant to give license to young diabetics or parents of young diabetics to be unconcerned about high blood sugars. I'm only referring to the years I had diabetes prior to the availability of self-testing. I certainly recommend good control from the start, but you should know that in at least one person's long-term diabetic experience high blood sugars at a young age turned out okay.

It's important for young people and parents of youngsters with diabetes to continue to be conscientious about maintaining reasonably normal blood sugars; however, if your youngster is a Type 1 diabetic, you are going to see blood sugars in the 300-to-400 range once in a while. The important reactions are to learn from each high episode. Correct them right away but don't burden yourself or your youngster with unnecessary anxiety.

Another little-discussed advantage that young people have when diabetes is diagnosed at an early age is the healthier eating habits they will develop out of necessity. These eating habits will limit weight gain and therefore limit future health problems that result from being overweight or obese. With the technology available now and with a desire to develop healthy eating and activity lifestyles, young diabetics today have a great chance, in my opinion, to live a healthier, longer life than many of their nondiabetic contemporaries.

High Blood Sugars at a Later Age

As I've said before, when young people get diabetes, their circulatory systems, and hearts are young and healthy. This means a longer grace period to learn all about diabetic control before any degenerative effects begin to develop, if at all. When an older person gets diabetes, it's often a result of some bad health habits developed over an extended period of time. When these bad habits begin, they can be compared to a thread that can pretty easily be broken. As bad habits continue, those threads develop into strings and then into ropes and become much harder to break. The older a person is when he or she develops diabetes, the naturally less resilient his or her body is and the less grace period he or she has to learn about diabetes and take the action needed to change habits. The difficulty of breaking bad habits combined with the shorter grace period gives Type 2 diabetics a more difficult task and a greater urgency to learn and adapt than Type 1 diabetics.

Is Blood Sugar Fluctuation the Culprit?

Type 1 diabetics may often hear people refer to the "fluctuation" of blood sugar as the cause of long-term complications. By my reasoning, if fluctuation were the problem, you'd be better off when you got a reading of 300 or higher just to leave it there and not cause fluctuation by bringing it down by 200 points to a more appropriate level. But fluctuation is not the main problem. The biggest problem is the frequency and more importantly the duration of the highs. So put fluctuation as a primary cause on the back burner when you're considering long-term complications. Remember, it's primarily the duration and frequency of the highs that will cause the problems. Every Type 1 diabetic is going to have blood sugars periodically in the 300s or even sporadically in the 400s. The key is responding promptly and appropriately and bringing it down to the more normal 75–105 range.

Type 2 diabetics will rarely see the extremely high blood sugars that a Type 1 may see periodically. But the problem for Type 2 diabetics is the more moderate high blood sugars—120 to 140—that may happen with some regularity and not be corrected.

In the balance of this book, you're going to learn how to mitigate or completely eliminate all these potential problems, and some Type 2 diabetics may eliminate diabetes altogether. If you don't have diabetes, you're going to learn how to reduce your chances of ever getting it by losing weight. You'll have the information to live healthier, happier, and longer. You can do it.

Chapter 3

The Very Best Medicine for Dealing with Type 1 or Type 2 Diabetes
A Positive Attitude

For all Type I and Type 2 diabetics, insulin-dependent or not; borderline diabetics, and prediabetics

Today I will be healthy, happy, productive, growing, and giving. My daily morning reminder to myself

—Rick Mystrom

Diabetes Shouldn't Dominate Your Life

It was April, 2004, about 40 years after my diagnosis as a diabetic. My family and I were in a small, beachfront restaurant in Lahaina on the island of Maui in Hawaii. My wife, Mary, and I had been married 34 years. Our oldest son, Nick, was 33, our son Rich was 30, and our daughter, Jen, was 27. Our family, including our soon-to-be son-in-law, Andy Scott, was on our almost annual vacation to Hawaii. We were eating lunch and I can't quite conjure up the reason for the comment, but my daughter, Jen, said, "Dad, you've never complained or made a big deal about having diabetes and that's made such a difference in our family

AUTHOR'S NOTE:

This chapter is so important some parts of it are included in my previous book, My Wonderful Life with Diabetes.

life." My son Rich, chipped in, "We all feel that way, Dad." Nick and Mary nodded in agreement.

The significance of that comment was that even though I had had diabetes for over 40 years, it was the first time I remember anyone really verbalizing the fact that I never complained about it.

My family had always been very supportive and helpful and I thought intuitively that they all felt I handled diabetes well. But the fact that it had never been verbalized was a testament to the fact that it was not a front- and-center issue in our family life. It was there but in the background. Mary and the kids were very aware of the immediate dangers of extreme low blood sugar and of the more subtle symptoms of moderately low blood sugar. If I seemed a little disjointed in my conversation or a little irritable (both of which are, by the way, symptoms of low blood sugar), the kids would ask if my blood sugar was low.

I wondered sometimes if it had been smart of me to tell the kids that low blood sugar made me irritable because that became the question they often asked if they thought I was being unfairly mad at them. "Dad, is your blood sugar low?" It made me stop and think that maybe my little irritation wasn't caused by them.

An Active Life

The point is that my having diabetes wasn't a dominant part of our family life and didn't keep us from doing whatever we wanted to do wherever we wanted to do it. As a family, we skied in Austria, Switzerland, Colorado, and Alaska. We Scuba-dived and snorkeled in Hawaii and the Caribbean. We went to water parks across America when the kids were young and as the kids got older, we water-skied in Arkansas, California, and Wisconsin. We took the kids to the Gobi Desert region in northern China in the middle of the winter. I took my two boys to Japan with a Little League team I coached to play against the Japanese kids. After we returned, Jen was prompted to say, "Dad, next time you go to Japan, can I go? I'm already seven years old and I haven't even been to Japan yet."

Now that the kids are grown and on their own, Mary and I have continued our world travels and activities: the Olympics in Athens in 2004, hiking down the Grand Canyon in 2006, and spending a month in Malawi in Central Africa to work at an orphanage in 2007. Closer to home, we downhill-ski, cross-country-ski, waterski, wake-surf, hike, bike, Rollerblade, play golf, and play tennis.

I credit a lot of my good health with diabetes to a lifetime of activity, but even if you haven't been active to this point, you will be surprised at how good you will feel—both mentally and physically—if you start increasing your physical activity.

Throughout this book, you'll find a theme of action, activity, and involvement. I recommend this active lifestyle to all diabetics. It's especially important for Type 2 diabetics.

Everyone will have his or her own capabilities and limits. But whether your activity is climbing mountains or climbing stairs, walking trails or walking malls, walking around the block or around your yard, playing sports or playing with your kids, my message is this: Get out and do what you can. Take part in whatever physical activity you're capable of.

Throughout this book, I'll be talking about activities, eating habits, and blood sugar control. Each chapter will add to your understanding of diabetes and to improvement of your life with diabetes. But remember this: Nothing is more important than a positive attitude toward diabetes and toward life in general.

The Mothers' Club and Their Secret to Long Lives

During my first term as mayor of Anchorage, Mary was invited to have tea one afternoon with a small group of ladies in Anchorage who called themselves "The Mothers' Club." But according to Mary, they were all grandmothers and many were great-grandmothers. Mary guessed that their average age was probably in the mid- to high 80s with a few in their low to mid-90s.

That night at dinner as Mary and I were talking, I asked her about her tea with the Mothers' Club. She said she'd had a delightful time. The ladies were all pleasant, positive, and friendly and all were very alert. She also reported that they all loved living in Anchorage and they thought that I was doing a great job as mayor. Not only that, but they thought that the mayor before me and the mayor before that had also done great jobs. In fact, they were pretty sure that every mayor in Anchorage's history had done a great job.

After they finished reminiscing and glowing about Anchorage, their children, their grandchildren, and life in general, Mary asked them the perfect question: "What do you attribute your long lives and good health to?" The answer surprised her. They all agreed that it was *a positive attitude*. That clearly explains why they thought every mayor in Anchorage's history had done a great job.

They all pretty much agreed that they weren't complainers, worriers, or critics. Rather, they saw themselves as being supportive, encouraging, and caring. They felt better because they made others feel better. That was their prescription for a long, happy life.

Every day in our lives, each of us has the opportunity to make others feel better, whether it's a server in a restaurant, a clerk in a retail store, or just someone you're passing on the sidewalk. A kind word, a compliment, or even just a smile that makes them feel better will make you feel better too—guaranteed. I've found that it's a lot easier to have a positive attitude about diabetes if you have a positive attitude about life.

As you're dealing with the challenges of making your life healthier with diabetes, you'll be happier if that isn't your total focus. Every chance you get, try to do some little, thoughtful deed for someone else. Each time you do, it will help put you in touch with your worth in life. And some of those little helpful deeds will always be remembered by the recipients and may then be passed forward to someone else.

It's easier to be positive about diabetes if you're also aware of trying to make your life better in other areas. My reminder to myself each morning in the shower is this simple statement: *"Today I'm going to be healthy, happy, productive, growing, and giving."* This reminds me every morning that I have to do what I can to maintain my health as a diabetic but it also reminds me that my life is full and diabetes is just one element.

The Special Importance of Attitude for Older Type 2 Diabetics

Type 2 diabetes is typically considered less serious than Type 1. The reasons are, on the surface, quite obvious. With Type 1 diabetes no insulin is produced and insulin injections or infusions are essential to survival. With Type 2 diabetes, some insulin is produced by the pancreas and oral medications can often normalize blood sugars by stimulating the production of more insulin. Not only can oral medications be effective with Type 2, but very often, a change in eating habits, loss of weight, and more physical activity can normalize blood sugar levels and preclude the need for either oral medication or insulin injections.

As I said in chapter 1, I believe that considering Type 2 diabetes less serious than Type 1 is a danger that very often leads to significant health problems and a shorter life for those Type 2 diabetics who don't very quickly develop an understanding and a positive approach to dealing with their challenge.

So why is Type 2 so serious and why is a positive attitude of special importance to older Type 2 diabetics? To start with, Type 2 diabetes usually develops in people over 40 years old and is much more common in people who are overweight. When Type 2 diabetes manifests itself in older people, it's usually a result of long-developing, at least moderately unhealthy eating habits, and a slowly diminishing level of activity.

In my personal observations and discussions, a significant number of older male Type 2 diabetics were active in athletics in their youth. With that high level of activity, they had the luxury of eating whatever they wanted, whenever they wanted, and as much as they wanted without the resulting weight gain that nonathletes would have experienced. But after the competitive activity in their lives stopped, their eating portions often did not change.

Two major issues are at play here: (1) Long-term bad habits are hard to break and, (2) when you get diabetes at a later age, your body is not as healthy and resilient as the bodies of those who may get Type 1 diabetes when they're much younger.

If you're an older Type 2 diabetic and you have habits to break, you must realize that you have a smaller window of time than a younger diabetic would have to change those habits. You can't take five or 10 years to change your habits and normalize your blood sugars.

Contrast that small window of time for a Type 2 diabetic with my personal experience having contracted Type 1 diabetes at age 20. I tried to learn everything I could about diabetes, but self-testing wasn't available. I was also not settled in one state for quite a few years after I was diagnosed, and I didn't have a regular doctor. Consequently, I knew what my blood sugars were only after the two or three times a year when I visited a doctor and had a lab test for blood sugar done. Then it took three days for the doctor to get the results from a lab. And quite frankly, they were often in the 200-to-300 mg/dl range. But because I was young, active, and healthy, I had quite a few years to learn how to control my blood sugars without much damage apparently done.

I have mentioned that the one problem I have as a result of having diabetes for 50 years is a diminished sensitivity in my feet called neuropathy. My podiatrist tells me that he feels that may be because of my high blood sugars at an early age. So although a younger person has a larger window of time to adapt, it shouldn't be interpreted as a total free ride.

I don't mean to imply that a young Type 1 diabetic should take a long time to adapt to having diabetes. With the current technology you can adapt to diabetes a lot faster than I did nearly 50 years ago.

But if it does take some time for young Type 1 diabetics to accept and adapt, it will probably harm them less than older Type 2 diabetics who take the same length of time to adapt. I know a half dozen people in Anchorage who contracted Type 2 diabetes in their 50s or early 60s and died within 10 to 12 years. That should not happen. Being diagnosed as a Type 2 diabetic at any age can be your ticket to a longer, healthier life—not a sentence to a shorter, unhealthy life. It's up to you. It's a wake-up call that says start now—don't wait.

Most Type 2 diabetics I talk to have a strong aversion to starting insulin injections. That's natural. But at some point, if improvements in eating habits, increases in physical activity, or taking oral medication all fail to normalize blood sugars, some method of insulin injection or infusion is not only necessary but also desirable. Most Type 2 diabetics who reach that point do settle into an injection routine that—after a short period of time— becomes comfortable and not too burdensome. They also tell me that they feel better, have more energy, and sleep better.

A positive attitude and a willingness to learn and act on what you learn can be your ticket to eliminating the symptoms of Type 2 diabetes or living a long, happy life with Type 2 diabetes. It's most important for you to consider being diagnosed as a Type 2 diabetic as an *opportunity* to live a longer, healthy life, not as a *sentence* to a shorter, unhealthy life.

A good place to start is to consider some promise to yourself.

Some Promises You Should Consider

Living a healthy, active life with diabetes starts with you. It starts with a promise. Here are some promises to consider as you go forward.

1. I accept the fact that I have diabetes. I know that I have to be a little smarter and a little more careful about what I eat than other people. I also know that if I test my blood appropriately,

I will know more about what foods will keep me healthy than nondiabetics will know. I will understand the impact of foods and exercise on my health and my weight.

2. I will develop good exercise and eating patterns that I will eventually turn into habits I can maintain. I recognize that neither my exercise nor my eating patterns will be perfect, but I know they don't have to be. They just have to be good.

3. I promise that I will not complain about having diabetes but that I will learn from it and if I apply what I learned, I know that I will feel better, be healthier, and be trimmer than most nondiabetics.

4. I promise that I will not let diabetes keep me from doing anything in the world that I want to do with my life. I know that if I keep this promise I can live a healthy, active, and fulfilling life with diabetes

That's a lot to think about, but keep referring to this chapter. If you can make and keep your own promise from these ideas, every day will dawn a little brighter.

As I've spoken to groups about diabetes and mentioned my promise never to complain about being a diabetic, it has become the single point that doctors in the audience have most often commented positively about. Their typical reaction is, "If I could get all my patients to think that way, they would be so much healthier." Attitude is, in my mind, the most important single factor in living with diabetes. If you can have or develop a good attitude about your diabetes and your life, you can live healthy, live well, and live long with diabetes.

Chapter 4

The Three Elements of a
Healthy Diabetes Lifestyle

*"Premera Blue Cross has been promoting health and wellness
for some years now, and according to Jeff Davis, Premera's
president, seventy-five percent of all health care spending
results from chronic diseases, like diabetes and heart disease,
which are heavily influenced by choices people make,
primarily smoking, poor diet, and lack of exercise."* [1]

A Clear Message from a Straight-Talking Doctor

A few winters ago at a reception celebrating Fur Rendezvous, Alaska's
traditional winter gathering and celebration, a friend of mine and
former Alaska state legislator, candidly revealed he was really worried.
He had been recovering from a debilitating snowmobile accident that
had immobilized him and forced him into two years of sedentary
living. Mike was 68 years old at the time. He's a big guy— about 6
foot 3, an athlete in his youth, and somewhat overweight before his
accident. But he said since the accident his weight had climbed to
over 300 pounds.

The day before our conversation, he had met with his doctor, John
Schwartz, a mutual friend. One of the questions Mike asked Dr. Schwartz
was what he could expect with regard to mobility in his 70s. The doctor's

---

1   *Anchorage Daily News*, March 14, 2010, Tim Bradner

answer was startling to Mike. Dr. Schwartz said, "I don't know, Mike. I don't have any patients in their 70s who are over 300 pounds." Mike persisted. "But doctor, what do you think my mobility will be like?" According to Mike, Dr. Schwartz said, "Let me say it one more time, Mike. I don't have any patients over 300 pounds who are in their 70s."

The message was blunt and crystal clear. Lose weight or don't expect to live much longer. That message is consistent with an examination of 57 studies involving 900,000 people who were followed for 10 to 15 years. The study determined that about 33 percent of Americans were obese. That obesity created a life-shortening effect of 10 years, about the same as smoking. Another 33 percent of Americans were simply overweight. According to the study, coauthor Gary Whitlock, an epidemiologist at Oxford, "Obesity causes heart disease and stroke by pushing up blood pressure, mucking up [he's British] blood cholesterol, and triggering diabetes."[2]

Introduction to Healthy Living Lifestyles

We all read and hear a lot about *diet* and *exercise*. Depending on the expertise or the experience of the authors or the television hosts or hostesses, one of the two often gets precedence over the other. And in almost all cases, any discussion on food will focus on diets which are typically unsustainable over a long period of time. Or if exercise is the subject, the focus will typically be an intense, structured exercise program, which is equally unsustainable. Because almost all of these intense diets and intense exercise programs are not regimens that can become lifestyles, put those concepts out of your mind as you read this book.

Lately, I've started talking to friends, acquaintances, and strangers about their eating, activity, and exercise habits. I've talked mostly to those who appear to be trim and in good shape because it's a lot harder to talk about lifestyle habits with folks who are not trim. Although

---

2   *USA Today*, March 18, 2009, Nancy Hellmich

most of the information on healthy lifestyles comes from my personal experience, I've found that these discussions have broadened my knowledge and confirmed many of my conclusions.

In this and future chapters, you'll be learning how to develop healthy eating, activity, and exercise lifestyles that can easily become part of your overall "healthy living lifestyle."

I use the word *lifestyle* as opposed to *diet* when I'm talking about food. Diets are often temporary eating actions to achieve a specific weight loss goal in a specific length of time. Most typically when that time is over old habits—and old weight—reappear. The eating lifestyle I'll be showing you is a pattern of eating that you will learn and that will become a habit in a surprisingly short time.

These three healthy lifestyles: eating, activity, and exercise are covered in more detail in later chapters. If you embrace these three lifestyles as patterns, they will soon transition to habits and improve your life, health, and happiness.

A Healthy Eating Lifestyle

Ask yourself how many times you've looked at a lean, trim person and thought, "How can she eat that much and stay thin?" Or maybe you've thought, "That guy never diets. I'm always dieting and I'm fatter than he is." And have you ever noticed that people who are lean or of normal weight are rarely dieting and people who are overweight seem to be dieting often or maybe always?

Why the incongruity? The answer is pretty simple. The people who are not overweight have developed an eating lifestyle they don't think much about anymore. It just happens. They do it by habit. Perhaps they learned the habits from their parents, maybe they sought out information on food, or maybe they just fell into that healthy eating lifestyle, but whatever the answer, you'll rarely hear them talk about it. They don't focus on food. They just eat the right foods and the right portions by habit. Though I said the answer was simple, I recognize that the solution is not so simple. Changing habits is always hard but this book is designed to make changing your habits much easier.

A Healthy Activity Lifestyle

What is a "healthy activity lifestyle"? What does that mean? Many of the leaner, fitter people I know and talk to, especially in their late 40s and older have more activity in their daily lives than their overweight counterparts do. It may or may not be structured motion but they just move a lot during their day. Most of the fit people I know who are in their late 70s or in their 80s and 90s don't claim any structured programs other than walking and just moving more than their over-weight counterparts. Most love walking and they say so.

A general activity or motion lifestyle can be developed whether you live in a city, or in suburbs or small towns, and the benefits will be tremendous. The biggest benefit of this lifestyle is that it will help you lose weight through your daily living. A secondary benefit that I've noted from my personal experience and from a study that I'll quote later is that people are less likely to snack when they're active than when they're sedentary.

A Healthy Exercise Lifestyle

If you're a Type 2 diabetic, starting an exercise lifestyle can change your life. I know! I know! Lots of authors have said this before. Thousands of books are available on becoming an aerobic running machine, developing abs that look like ski moguls, or creating a butt that stops traffic as you pass by. None of that is bad but the problem is those results are not going to happen without devoting a big part of your life to reaching those plateaus.

When I talk about a healthy exercise lifestyle, I'm talking about a pattern of exercise that you can follow the rest of your life, a pattern that will become a fun, comfortable part of your life, improve your muscle-to-fat ratio, improve your appearance, and improve your health.

I'll be talking about consistency over intensity and moderation over maximization. Two bits of advice I'll be talking about are first, "Don't work too hard," because if you do you won't continue and second, "Throw the whole idea of 'no pain, no gain' in the trash can of bad advice." Working too hard if you're not accustomed to it will likely end with muscle and tendon injuries and feeling that you can't gain without pain will just discourage you from continuing. It's too hard and no fun.

By gradually adding more muscle in a moderate but continuing exercise lifestyle, you will naturally burn more fat more easily. That will make your continuing weight loss through your healthy eating and active lifestyles easier to maintain.

In this book I'll be talking not only about moderation in eating, but more importantly, about eating the right foods; I'll be talking not only about moderation in exercise, but also about adding a gradually increasing activity level to your life.

The Relative Importance of the Three Factors: Eating, Activity, and Exercise

After living with diabetes for nearly 50 years and testing my blood sugar an estimated 60,000 times after eating, after exercise, and after activities, I have very specific and measurable information about the importance of each of these three factors.

A *healthy eating lifestyle* is unequivocally the most important factor in a healthy life. Now that we've put the word *diet* aside and are thinking instead of a *healthy eating lifestyle,* you'll want to develop the right patterns of eating that will in time become your habits. You'll soon understand what those patterns are and how they can become habits. The second most important element of a healthy life is creating the habit of putting more motion in your daily life. Doing that doesn't mean changing your life. It simply means noticing and taking advantage of the dozens of opportunities around you every day to move a little more, burn more glucose, while giving yourself less opportunity to snack. I'm talking about walking, doing yard work, doing housework, getting to know your neighborhood from a pedestrian perspective, parking a few extra blocks away from restaurants or work, playing with the kids or grandkids more, riding a bike more often if you can. An *active lifestyle* is the second most important factor in a healthy life. In Chapter 10 I'll give you techniques for simply and enjoyably adding activity to your daily life.

The third factor in the health equation is a structured exercise program. This is the least important of the three factors but still important. I would describe it as desirable but not necessary. A moderate exercise program means reserving some time three to six days a week—you choose—to create your own exercise routine from the structure I provide. The key to this program is "Don't ever work so hard that you don't want to do it again." It's all about consistency, not intensity. In chapter 11 I'll explain the program that has worked well for me and can work well for you.

So here's the formula. Healthy living means eating the right foods, having physical activity in your lifestyle, and adding moderate but sustainable exercise.

I'm not advocating perfection or intensity in any of these factors. The key to *healthy eating* is not continually pushing away foods you like or giving up all desserts forever. A healthy eating lifestyle is simply understanding what foods are the biggest contributors to weight gain and minimizing those foods and what foods contribute least to weight gain or most to weight loss and maximizing those foods.

How Can I, as a Type 1 Diabetic, Measure the Relative Importance of Food, Motion, and Exercise— and Why Can Only a Type 1 Do This?

Exercise and motion are both important for good health. No doubt about it. I've had a moderate, structured exercise program for about 15 years now—pretty consistent in the winter, not so much in the summer. Before that I had been very active in recreational and competitive sports but didn't have a regular exercise program. But how can I tell that exercise and motion are less important than healthy eating in terms of blood sugar control and losing weight? These next few pages will explain how I can tell.

After my first two years as mayor of Anchorage, I realized I was getting a little softer around the middle and a little smaller in the chest and shoulders. I had slipped in my standard way of measuring my muscular fitness, which is to have an 8- to 10-inch difference between my jacket size and my waist size. For example, a size 44 jacket and 34-inch waist for pants is good for me. A 44 jacket and 36-inch waist is not quite as good. A 42 jacket and 38-inch waist would be even worse. The 8- to 10-inch "jacket size to pants size rule" is a good guide for most guys. It's a better way to look at general body composition than the Body Mass Index concept because you don't get penalized for being more muscular than average. If you have a 10-inch or greater jacket-over-waist-size, you're doing just fine.

Maybe right now your jacket-size-to-pants-size ratio may be reversed. Maybe you're looking at a 44 jacket and 46-inch waist or maybe a 48 jacket and 54-inch waist. Don't be discouraged—things will change based on what you're about to learn. I wish I had a similar formula for women's dress and waist sizes, but since this is based on my personal experience, I don't. But everything else in this book relates to both men and women.

Toward the end of my first term, my wife, Mary, while attending a Covenant House fundraiser, won some physical training sessions with Anchorage resident and fitness trainer Philip Bradfield, who had recently won a National Master's Bodybuilding Championship. Philip worked at the Alaska Club, the fitness center Mary and I were members of.

Mary started working a little with Philip and gave me good reports so I decided to try using Philip as a trainer. Philip's not a big guy but boy, did he have a good physique. He was the first person under 175 pounds to win the National Master's Open Championship while competing as a lightweight. After meeting Philip, one of the first questions I asked was his jacket size and his waist size. I was just checking to see if he met my 10-inch difference standard. He said, "My jacket size is 44 and my waist is 30 inches, but I'm not training." It was almost as if he was apologizing for his extraordinarily good 14-inch difference between jacket size and waist size.

Philip was very knowledgeable and comfortable to work with and has since become a friend. He got me started on a track of regular workouts which I address in later chapters. But it was something he said on the first day that I never forgot. He said, "Mayor, long-term fitness is 80 percent diet* and 20 percent exercise"—this from a guy who made his living teaching people how to properly exercise. I initially gave a cursory nod of agreement but didn't really buy into it then.

AUTHOR'S NOTE:

What Philip was referring to when he used the word diet was general eating patterns or habits, not a specific short-term "lose weight fast" diet.

Well, over the past 15 years I've come around to knowing that eating is more important than exercise in losing and maintaining a desirable weight and good health. I don't know if healthy eating is exactly 80 percent of the equation, but thousands of blood sugar tests over the past 10 years have convinced me that 80 percent is pretty close. I'm now certain that the fuel I put in my body plays a much bigger part in determining my weight and health than how I burn that fuel.

So how have I come to agree with Philip about the much greater role of food than of the other two elements?

To understand how I can tell, it's important to recall that insulin is the hormone that allows the body to use energy and store fat. The more glucose that enters the bloodstream, the more insulin is triggered and enters the bloodstream. As more insulin is triggered it means more weight is gained. So when I say something triggers more insulin demand, that means more weight gain or less weight loss. Conversely, less insulin demand means less weight gain or more weight loss. This is true for everyone. The only difference between me, as an insulin-dependent Type 1 diabetic, and most others is that I get a report each day from my insulin pump telling me how much insulin I took that day to balance the food I ate. It's like a daily report card on the impact of food, motion, and exercise on my weight and health.

Here's how I arrived independently at roughly the same percentages Philip stated on my first visit with him. On days that I don't follow my normal healthy eating patterns but am active and follow my exercise program, my insulin demand will typically go from 30 units a day on a healthy eating day to about 42 units or more on that bad eating day. That's an increase of 12 units of insulin demand. On days that I do follow my healthy eating patterns but don't move much and don't do my structured exercise program, my insulin demand will go up about 3 units. So a day without much motion and little or no structured exercise will increase my insulin demand by 3 units while a bad eating day will raise my insulin demand by 12 units. That's four times more than the other two elements combined—right at Philip's ratio of 80 to 20 percent.

I've had an insulin pump that gives me these daily reports of insulin taken for about 10 years now. These daily reports continue to support my conclusion that healthy eating is about 80 percent of healthy living and weight control and an active lifestyle plus a regular exercise program are about 20 percent. By a ratio of 4 to 1, what you put into your body is more important than how you burn it. Another way to state this very important premise is that an unhealthy eating day even with activity and exercise will contribute about four times more fat to your body than a healthy eating day with little or no exercise and motion.

Keep in mind there are certainly exceptions to this ratio, especially for competitive athletes who are engaged in intensive training programs; but for the majority of Americans I believe this ratio applies.

When I was working out with Philip, I noticed many people, men and women, who seemed to be working much harder than I was. Some were very committed to their schedule of hard strength and aerobic workouts but even after watching them each morning for a few weeks or more I didn't notice any apparent results of their hard work. I asked Philip about that and he said simply, "They're not eating right. They can't gain muscle if they don't eat enough protein."

Another conclusion I've come to after observing others in gyms over the years is that those who work too hard don't last. Hence my philosophy of not working so hard that you don't want to come back the next day.

In summary, you can lose weight with good eating habits and bad activity and exercise habits; but you can't lose weight with good activity and exercise habits and bad eating habits. People can get stronger and more aerobically fit with exercise alone but if eating habits are bad, the best anyone can do is get fit, fat, and strong. A more likely scenario if you don't have good eating habits is the "fit" part goes away and you're left with fat and strong.

Good Eating Habits, an Active Lifestyle, and Good Exercise Habits Work Together to Support Each Other

Now that I've put eating patterns out in front, I also have to say I am a big believer in both an active lifestyle and a structured, moderate exercise program. Those three friends of good health, *good eating habits, a generally active lifestyle, and a moderate exercise program* work together to steadily bring health and satisfaction to your life.

In defense of wanting you to develop all three of these habits or lifestyles, I have three early observations to share.

First, eating well and exercising support each other psychologically. On days when I exercise, I'm more likely to follow good eating patterns because I don't want to waste the potential muscle gain by eating badly. Conversely, when I have a good healthy eating day with plenty of protein, I don't want to waste that by not working out. The two support and encourage each other. As an aside, muscle gain is as important for women as it is for men. A higher percentage of muscle for both men and women means better posture, better coordination, better circulation, and more efficient fat burning, as you'll learn in my second observation.

My second observation in defense of exercise is this. Like many other people, I've had stages in my life when I've been more muscular and stages when I've been less muscular. When I'm at a more muscular stage I require less insulin for the same foods and portion sizes than I do at the less muscular stages of my life. That supports the axiom that muscle tissue burns more calories than fat tissue. Muscle tissue is very active, continually contracting and expanding. Every pound of muscle you add to your body means you'll burn about 50 to 100 calories a day more than if you were to add a pound of fat. If you lose weight by diet alone, you will be losing both muscle and fat, which will make it harder to continue or maintain your loss.

In other words, a more muscular person can eat the same amount of food as a less muscular person of the same weight and not gain as much weight. Whether you're a man or woman, the more muscle tissue you have, the more you become a fat-burning machine.

My third observation presented itself to me while writing my two books on diabetes. The past three winters I've spent researching and writing these books have been the least physically active winters of my life. I'm still pretty consistently going to the gym for my regular, moderate workouts. But I'm still spending much, much more time sitting at my computer than I ever have. That inactivity, I've discovered, creates a great opportunity and tendency to snack.

Most of my snacks are pretty healthy: usually smoked salmon, celery, broccoli, cauliflower, and carrots, most of the time dipped in blue cheese dressing—which you'll learn later is not a problem under certain conditions. Blueberries are also one of my favorites as are cashews and almonds. But I'm also susceptible to a handful of potato chips, maybe an Oreo or two, and rice crackers or Swedish hard bread with butter (one of my favorites). Maybe once a month I'll have a small bowl of ice cream—but rarely in the evening and never just before going to bed. (You'll read more on that timing later).

My point is *inactivity and a more sedentary life encourage and promote snacking. Activity discourages snacking.*

What about Gastric Bypass Surgery for the Obese?

I've included this story about Carol White, a friend of mine and a Type 2 diabetic, for two reasons: first, to illustrate that healthy eating is the most important factor in weight reduction and it can be achieved solely by changing eating habits. But in Carol's case she used a more dramatic method. By now you know I don't recommend trying to lose weight only by eating habits without adding motion and exercise but it can be done. In Carol's case she did it. But in her case she also recognizes that to stay healthy she needs to add motion and a moderate exercise program to her life.

The second reason I'm including Carol's story is the beautifully descriptive way she recounts the results of her weight loss and the positive effect weight loss had on her health and self-esteem.

Before I say anything else about Carol's success, I need to clarify that she had a Roux-en-Y gastric bypass surgery to limit the size of her stomach. Bariatric surgery, in general, takes a number of forms and I'm neither recommending nor discouraging anyone from using this method. However, this surgery is gaining traction as an option for Type 2 diabetics. It has proven to be successful in bringing Carol's Type 2 diabetes into remission.

Carol White's Story

A few years ago at an Alaska Sports Hall of Fame press conference held by our board of directors, I noticed a lady in the audience who

I felt I knew but I couldn't place her. After the event was over, I walked up to her, apologized for not knowing who she was, and asked her name. She said "Carol White." I was stunned. Over the past half dozen years I had sat next Carol and talked with her at a dozen or so West Anchorage High School basketball games, a team her brother, Chuck White, coached with great success. I've known her casually for maybe 20 years. During that time Carol was a pleasant lady, easy to talk with, who had steadily gained weight over 25 years and consequently developed Type 2 diabetes.

She is now slim, attractive, and very healthy looking. She has gone from 284 pounds on November 2, 2010 to 150 pounds on the day I saw her at the press conference, December 5, 2011—an extraordinary loss of 134 pounds in 13 months.

Here is the clear and beautiful way Carol describes the change in her life as a result of her weight loss:

> "I had surgery November 2, 2010. The only regret I have is that I didn't find Dr. Afram sooner and have the surgery years ago. I'd been overweight for at least 25 years, was **Type 2 diabetic** [Carol's emphasis], had high blood pressure, high cholesterol, was using a C-pap machine to combat sleep apnea, and was generally without energy. Sluggish was my 'normal' speed of progressing through life.

> "Prior to my surgery I was taking nine different prescription medications for various ailments. Today I take one low-dose prescription once a day to maintain my current blood pressure, which I suspect I'll be able to stop taking soon. Plus I take bariatric vitamins!

> "It's been one year since my surgery and I have been off my diabetes medication since just a few days after my surgery. My blood sugar

*is NORMAL [all caps are her emphasis]. My cholesterol is
EXCELLENT. My blood pressure is NORMAL and I've been off
my C-pap machine for sleep apnea since about 5 months after the
surgery. I have energy and a zest for life that had been absent for
too long. I have lost 130 pounds in one year and have gone from a
woman's size 24 to a trim and SASSY size 8!! I'm literally half the
woman I used to be and couldn't be happier to say so!!*

*"I've been blessed with the support of my children and the
encouragement of friends, but ultimately the end results are up to
you. As someone who's 'been there, done that,' trust me when I
tell you, YOU CAN DO IT!"*

Carol White
Anchorage, Alaska

On March 24, 2012, I was a speaker at the highly successful annual
Diabetes Day event sponsored by the Rockwood Clinic in Spokane,
Washington. I was scheduled to speak at two of the sessions with an
hour break between them. During the break, I strolled across the hallway
and sat in on a talk being given by Dr. Carol Wysham with the Diabetes
and Endocrinology Center at the clinic. Dr. Wysham was the first medical
professional I had heard speak of bariatric surgery as a possible and
often successful option for treating Type 2 diabetes.

Three days later upon returning home to Anchorage, I saw a headline
in the *Anchorage Daily News* boldly stating, "Weight-loss surgery
beats medicine in diabetes fight." The story had originally been written
by Denise Grady for *The New York Times* on March 26, 2012. The
article refers to two studies recently published online by the *New
England Journal of Medicine*. The two studies, one by the Catholic
University in Rome and the other by the Cleveland Clinic, both
compared two types of bariatric surgery with medical treatment and

both showed the surgical option had better remission rates after one year than medical treatment.

More recently, a study published in *Diabetes Care*, July 2012 is referred to in *Diabetes Forecast* in September, 2012 under the headline: "Gastric Bypass for the Less Obese." Here's the entire content of that reference in *Diabetes Forecast*.

> "Studies have shown that gastric bypass surgery in severely obese people (those with a body mass index over 35) often results in remission of Type 2 diabetes. But few trials have focused on people at the lower end of the obesity range. That's why researchers studied 66 people with Type 2 diabetes with BMIs between 30 and 35. Each underwent Roux-en-Y gastric bypass surgery without complications (there are health risks with this surgery). After 6 years, 88 percent of the participants had full diabetes remission—an A1C under 6.5 percent without medication—and 11 percent had such improvement in blood glucose levels that they could dramatically reduce their diabetes medications. (Only one person didn't improve.) What's more, the surgery reduced participants' risk factors for cardiovascular disease, such as high blood pressure and high LDL ('bad') cholesterol."

I know a few people who have taken this path and for some it has worked well, for others it has not. To make it work you still must change what you eat, when you eat and how often you eat. It's a personal choice that requires a lot of research and discussion with a qualified doctor. A less traumatic and very effective long-term choice, in my opinion, is the healthy lifestyle changes I'm recommending in this book.

My point of including Carol's story is this. She lost the weight with little or no change in activity patterns or exercise. It was all in changing her eating patterns and portion size. Although she was forced to eat smaller portions because of her smaller stomach, she was not forced to eat the healthy foods that made her weight loss journey successful.

She told me she had done some water aerobics before her surgery but because she had to wear a band around her stomach for six months after the surgery, she couldn't do water aerobics during that time. She had done some walking before the surgery and as she began to lose weight she was able to do slightly more. Aside from her slight increase in walking, this loss was all eating pattern changes.

Carol is obviously very happy with her results but she also told me that she now has added activity to her lifestyle and intends to start a regular exercise program to build muscle and tone her body. She'll be more successful at keeping her weight off and firming her body by adding those two factors to her lifestyle.

The changes in eating, activity, and exercise patterns that you'll find in this book may not result in a loss of 134 pounds in the first year, like Carol's. But if you follow my advice you will begin to lose weight right away and that weight loss will continue until you reach your desired weight. But even before you reach that ideal weight point you'll start looking better and feeling better. You'll notice it yourself first but it won't be long before others notice it.

Most important, by adopting the three lifestyle changes in this book, maintaining your weight will not be a constant struggle, it will just happen because of your healthy lifestyles.

The next five chapters deal with the most important of the three elements essential to losing weight and becoming healthier—*food and eating patterns.*

SECTION
II

You've Got Diabetes—
Or Might Get Diabetes—
What Should You Eat?

For Type 2, Type 1, and Borderline Diabetics and Prediabetics … and Any Overweight Person Who Wants to Lose Weight

This section provides the essential background for Type 1 diabetics to better understand the impact of different foods on their blood sugar and improve their blood sugar control. For Type 2 diabetics, it provides the background information to understand how to lower blood sugar, lose weight, and eliminate the symptoms of diabetes. It will teach prediabetics or borderline diabetics how to avoid ever getting diabetes. This section will show nondiabetics how to lose weight and avoid ever getting diabetes.

And for all of the above—it will help you make healthy decisions for the rest of your lives.

Chapter 5

How We Get Fat

The best action *Type 1 diabetics* can take to improve blood sugar control and pave the way to a healthier, happier life is to understand the relationships of foods and insulin to blood sugar control. That understanding begins with this primer on food from a diabetic's perspective. By the time you finish this book, you'll have the information and understanding you need to normalize your blood sugars (and lose weight if that's your goal).

The best action *Type 2 diabetics* can take to avoid or eliminate the need to inject insulin and/or take oral medications is to lose weight and keep it off. The end result is a healthier, happier, longer life. By the time you finish this chapter, you'll have the information and understanding you need to lower your blood sugar and start losing weight. But more important, you'll learn how to stay at that new lower weight and maintain normal blood sugar for the rest of your life.

For most Type 2 diabetics, avoiding or eliminating the need for insulin injections is a high priority and evidence of dietary success. Most of the time, avoiding insulin injections is a very appropriate and healthy goal, but not always. Some Type 2 diabetics will feel better, have more energy and live healthier *with* daily injections. By following the path provided by this book, the vast majority of Type 2 diabetics will be able to avoid or eliminate the need for insulin injections. But if you're not one of those, don't be discouraged. You'll soon find a daily injection to be as simple and as natural as brushing your teeth. And with a positive attitude, your daily moment of pain won't hurt any more than a pinch and will disappear just as fast. And most important, you'll have more energy and feel better.

Weight Gain and the Type 2 Diabetic Epidemic

The most commonly used estimate of the number of Type 2 diabetics in the United States is 30 million, compared to about 3 million Type 1 diabetics. Many argue that the rate of increase of Type 2 diabetes puts it in the category of an epidemic, although unlike other more infamous epidemics such as the bubonic plague, influenza, cholera, and smallpox, it doesn't pose the likelihood of immediate death. It does, however, pose the likelihood of a significantly shortened lifespan for more people worldwide than any of its more infamous epidemic cousins.

Not only will unchecked Type 2 diabetes significantly shorten life span, but the precursors to diabetes, "prediabetes" and "borderline diabetes," will have already started the life-shortening process. High blood pressure and its offspring, heart disease, may be already evident. When you consider that the most common symptom of a heart attack is sudden death, the time to correct Type 2 diabetes or its precursors is today.

How important is weight in this epidemic? First, not all Type 2 diabetics are overweight and not all overweight people have Type 2 diabetes. Type 2 diabetes may in some cases be hereditary and may in many cases be culturally influenced, but clearly the most common characteristic of Type 2 diabetics is being overweight. Consequently, losing weight is the most prescribed action for Type 2 diabetics to take. Almost all Type 2 diabetics would like to lose weight. To do that, it's important to understand how we gain weight.

The Role of Insulin in Weight Gain or Loss

The decision maker in weight gain or loss is *insulin*. It has often been called "nature's fat traffic light" because it directs the glucose in your bloodstream to be used either for energy, to be stored in the liver as glycogen, or to be stored around your body as fat. It works the same for diabetics and non-diabetics but diabetics may have to stimulate the pancreas to provide sufficient insulin or they may have to add insulin themselves with shots or a pump.

In everyday language here's how insulin determines whether or not you will get fat. When you eat a meal that includes say, protein, any type of carbohydrates, and some fat; all of that food will be converted to some amount of glucose and show up in your bloodstream as blood sugar or blood glucose. (Remember I use those terms interchangeably in this book). When the glucose shows up in your bloodstream your pancreas receives a signal to produce insulin. That insulin is the hormone that will allow some of the glucose to get into cells as energy which we all need to function. After the energy need is satisfied, the excess glucose then goes to the liver to be stored as glycogen for short term storage and if even more excess glucose is available, it then goes to fat cells as long term fat storage. That's what shows up around your organs and your body as fat—in all the places you don't want it.

AUTHOR'S NOTE:

The four pages of this sub-section are critical to your understanding of how you raise or lower your blood sugar and how you gain or lose weight. Please read these pages over and over until you're confident that you fully understand this fundamental concept of weight gain or loss.

So the question is then, "what determines which glucose is used as energy and which is stored as fat?"

That determination is largely a function of *how much* glucose is entering your bloodstream and *how fast* it's entering. If more glucose is going into your bloodstream than is needed to provide energy for your daily activities the remainder will be stored. As you now know your body's first choice for storage—after its energy need is filled—is in the liver as glycogen. That glycogen will become a readily available source of energy in case you don't eat again for a number of hours. The second choice for storing what additional glucose you don't need is around your body as fat.

Those are the choices for storage. The choices for usage follow the same pattern. Your body will always choose the easiest source of energy first so available glucose in your bloodstream will always be the first to be used. If you need more energy than the available glucose will provide then your body will tap its second choice—glycogen from the liver which is also easily returned to your blood stream. Only when both of those choices are insufficient will your body call on its third choice—fat stored in and around your organs and body. That fat will be used for energy only when the other two sources are depleted, but—and this is a big but (no pun intended)—fat molecules are very stable and hard to break down and reconvert to energy. Thus, it's very hard for your body to use that fat. That's an important reason why losing existing fat can be so hard—but it can be done so don't despair.

So now we're coming to a conclusion that is very critical to your understanding the importance of the graphs you'll see in chapter 6 and why the amount of glucose created by different foods is important to you.

By controlling the amount of glucose going into your bloodstream, you can control the amount of insulin that will go into your bloodstream. And by controlling the amount of insulin, you can control your weight gain or weight loss. Less insulin going into your blood means weight loss; more insulin going into your bloodstream means weight gain. Hence the reason some refer to insulin as natures traffic light. So reducing the amount of insulin going into your bloodstream is the key to weight loss. **Remember you reduce the amount of insulin that goes into your bloodstream by controlling the amount of glucose going into your bloodstream**.

Lowering the glucose entering your bloodstream will give you three

AUTHOR'S NOTE:

This is so important I'll repeat it once more.

In order to lower your blood sugars and lose weight, you must reduce the amount of glucose and therefore insulin entering your blood stream. This is an absolutely critical point to lock into your mind.

very important results. *First,* the less glucose you put in your bloodstream, the more you will require your body to use glycogen from your liver and use the fat you have stored around your body. Second, less glucose in your blood stream means your pancreas will produce less insulin; and less insulin means less fat storage and less weight gain or more weight loss. And third, by keeping your glucose lower, you can postpone or avoid completely all the devastating complications from poorly controlled diabetes that I discussed in chapter 2.

So now you know that in order to control your weight and your health you must control your glucose. Insulin may be the "fat decision-maker" but too much glucose is the villain. Periodically I'll see books referring to too much *insulin* as the cause of weight gain. Insulin is really just the responder. Excess glucose is the cause and creator of fat.

The preceding paragraphs are critically important for both Type 1 and Type 2 diabetics to understand. I would not be overstating if I were to say to all diabetics that understanding your blood glucose levels and committing to keeping those levels more normal is going to make the difference between living a long, healthy life or a short, unhealthy life.

It's also very important for all diabetics to understand *how fast* different foods and combinations of foods impact blood sugar levels. Some foods convert to glucose much faster than others. If any foods cause your blood glucose to rise faster than you can burn it, the remainder will be stored in the liver as glycogen or around your body as fat. Foods that enter your blood stream as glucose more slowly allow you to use more of that glucose before it gets stored. So it's important for all diabetics to understand not only the amount of the blood glucose increase that a given food or combination of foods cause but also the speed of that increase. Both the size of the blood sugar increase and the speed are contributors to weight gain.

Whether you're a Type 1 diabetic, a Type 2 diabetic, pre-diabetic, borderline diabetic or non-diabetic; the more glucose you cause to enter your bloodstream, the more insulin your body will need and the end result of more insulin is more weight gain.

Using myself as an example, if what I've eaten over a period of a month produces an amount of glucose that requires me to give myself an average of about 36 units a day of insulin, I will gain weight during that month. If the food I've eaten over a month requires only an average of about 28 units of insulin a day, I will lose weight.

From 30 to 34 units of insulin a day is a generally stable range for my weight maintenance. Any weight gain or loss in that range will be pretty small and influenced by how active I might be during that period of time. These numbers will be different for different people but my point here is if you reduce your insulin demand and you will lose weight.

So how do you lower glucose, reduce insulin demand, and lose weight? You need to know what to eat.

Knowing *What* to Eat

Now you know that you should be lowering the amount of glucose that you're causing to enter your bloodstream. The logical question is, what foods will do that? How can you determine what foods will cause the highest or fastest blood sugar increases and what foods will cause the lowest or slowest increases—and what about all the foods in between?

By now you know that all foods—not just sweets—cause some rise in blood sugar. Protein, fats, vegetables, fruits, starches, and sweets all contribute some amount to your glucose level. So how do you find out which foods raise blood glucose fast and much and which foods don't? And every bit as important, which combinations of foods raise blood sugar fast and which don't.

What I've learned about foods from over 60,000 blood tests will provide the answers to help you better control and lower your blood sugar, lose weight, be healthier, and live longer. It took me 30 years to learn what foods and combinations of foods will best lower blood sugar and reduce weight. You'll learn it in a few short days.

As I've previously noted, for the past 30 years I've been testing my blood sugar before and after almost every meal. I've tested at least once and lately twice before I go to bed each night and after I wake up each morning. I also test before physical activities and many times after these activities. I also test at any other time I think my blood sugar needs adjusting. As a result of all these tests, I've learned how hundreds of different foods and combinations of foods will impact blood sugar and weight. I've learned not only *how much* different foods will raise my blood sugar—and yours as well—but also *how fast* those foods will raise my blood sugar.

It bears repeating that *how much* foods will raise your blood sugar and *how fast* foods will raise your blood sugars are both very important to your good health.

Which Foods Cause the Greatest Rise in Blood Sugar and the Greatest Gains in Weight and Which Will Not? And How Do I Know?

When Type 1 diabetics, such as I am, eat foods and cause glucose to enter the bloodstream, it cannot be used or stored naturally because no insulin is produced. The glucose simply collects in the bloodstream and causes a rise in blood sugar. This, of course, is why Type 1 diabetics need to inject the appropriate amount of insulin manually or with an insulin pump. But if I, as a Type 1 diabetic, eat food and *don't inject* insulin, I can measure exactly how much that food, or any food combination, makes my blood sugar rise. A big rise indicates a big contribution to weight gain and a smaller rise indicates a smaller contribution to weight gain. The less my blood sugar rises, the less insulin I need to inject and the smaller the contribution to weight gain or the bigger contribution to weight *loss*.

Why Only a Type 1 Diabetic Can Accurately Test the Impact of Food on Blood Sugar

Only a Type 1 diabetic can directly and accurately test foods' impact on blood sugar. That is exactly what I've done for this book. Although I've tested my blood sugar and generally analyzed the results for over 30 years, for the purpose of this book, I've specifically tested and graphed over 100 different foods or combinations of foods and not given myself any insulin for 90 minutes. Then I've tested my blood sugar (glucose) every 10 minutes during that time to determine how much and how fast each food or combination of foods has raised my blood sugar. This will provide—never before published—firsthand information for diabetics to improve control of their blood sugar and lose weight.

Type 2 diabetics cannot accurately test this way since their pancreas produces some—but usually not enough—insulin and therefore even as they eat food and increase their blood sugar, their pancreas is producing some insulin and decreasing blood sugar concurrently. That partial production of insulin negates their ability to measure the exact impact of foods on their blood sugar.

Nondiabetics cannot test foods' impact on blood sugar because for them the pancreas is working properly and producing sufficient insulin to use or store their glucose automatically as it enters the bloodstream.

Consequently, their blood sugar levels never rise like a diabetic's does, and a measurement of impact of specific foods is impossible. It's important to remember that even if a nondiabetic's blood sugar doesn't show a rise, the glucose is still going in and being stored, so the impact on weight gain is still happening.

That leaves only Type 1 diabetics able to get an accurate measure of the impact of foods on blood glucose. Less than 1 percent of America's population is a Type 1 diabetic but that's still a lot of folks, so why hasn't some other Type 1 done this?

First of all, a person who is going to do this would have to have a long history of testing and analysis to even begin. Maybe some people in the United States have tested blood sugars more than I have but I'm guessing that number is pretty small—maybe only a handful. I, of course have not graphed all the data I learned from 30 years of blood sugar testing. But whenever I measured, I would recall what I had most recently eaten and what activities I engaged in. After years of doing that I developed a clear understanding of the impact of different foods and food combinations. But the challenge for me in writing this book was how to represent that information graphically.

Three years ago I started testing and measuring foods—and drinks—and graphing the results to illustrate all these foods' impact on blood sugar and therefore weight.

To create these graphs I had to be willing to make a health sacrifice—although I'm confident it's a small sacrifice. I had to be willing to eat hundreds of different foods and not take any insulin for 90 minutes. That is the only way I know to illustrate the impact of foods and combinations of foods on my blood sugar. I have never seen or read any information about anyone who has actually tested the impact of foods this way.

To my knowledge, this type of human testing has never been previously published or perhaps even done. Researchers would be naturally hesitant to solicit diabetics to test this way because it involves the subjects' eating various foods and not taking insulin for some period of time. This is not a healthy action for diabetics. I did it because I believe quantifying and graphing this information and combining it with what I have learned over the past 30 years of multiple daily blood tests, will help millions of diabetics have healthier, happier, longer lives.

I've been absorbing this information about what foods normalize my blood sugars and moderate my need for insulin for over 30 years now by continual blood sugar testing. I've come to some very important, generalized information that has served me well and I believe helped thousands of diabetics who have attended presentations I have made over the years. The specific tests I have done for this book have not only ratified most of my findings, but have also clarified some issues that had been perplexing to me.

A Key Point to Remember

As you read this chapter and review the graphs, remember this: insulin is the key that opens the passageway for the glucose in the bloodstream to be sent to cells to be burned as energy, to be sent to the liver to be stored as glycogen, or to be sent to fat cells to be stored as fat. In short, the foods that raise your blood sugar the most will require the most insulin to be produced by your body or injected and will contribute the most to weight gain. The foods that raise your blood sugar the least will make your blood sugar easier to control and contribute the least to weight gain or will cause weight loss.

The foods you eat cannot be used as energy without insulin. They cannot be stored in your liver without insulin, and cannot be stored as fat around your body without insulin. Every person's weight gain (diabetic or not) is directly related to the amount of insulin produced by the body or self-injected.

Do Some People Need High-Glucose-Creating Foods?

Yes. Some people need to eat foods that generate the *most* blood glucose and therefore the highest insulin demand. Who are they?

The first group who should eat these foods is that tiny percentage of adult Americans who actually want to gain weight. If you're one of that relatively small group, the place to start is the Department of Agriculture Food Pyramid. It provides an excellent summary of how to gain weight fast without eating a lot of sweets. The other people who need more high-glucose-producing foods than I will be recommending are active children, active teens, and competitive athletes. They need easily accessible energy and will burn most of the glucose created by these foods before it gets a chance to be stored as fat.

A Quick Review of Why This Information about Food Applies to Type 2, Type 1, Prediabetics, and Borderline Diabetics as well as Nondiabetics

For Type 2 diabetics, how much different foods raise your blood sugar is important because, as you now know, the more a food raises your blood sugar, the greater the demand for insulin. More insulin (whether you inject it or your pancreas produces it) means more weight gain. So when I talk about certain foods that will significantly raise your blood sugar, what follows is that these foods will require more insulin and contribute significantly to weight gain. Watch out for them.

For Type 2 diabetics also, how fast foods will raise your blood sugar is very important. You now know that if certain foods raise your blood sugar faster than you need it, the unused glucose will be stored first in your liver and later around your body. That's bad. That means weight gain. But if certain foods raise your blood sugar at about the same speed or more slowly than you burn it, those calories can be used before they are stored. That's good. That means weight stability or weight loss.

For Type 1 diabetics, both how much and how fast certain foods will make your blood sugar go up are also very important. Knowing those two factors and being able to predict the action of foods (or liquids) will help immensely in your ability to anticipate and control your blood sugar levels.

For nondiabetics the same issues are important. If any foods enter your bloodstream as glucose *faster* than your body needs it, the excess will be stored. If those foods create more glucose than you need, that excess will also be stored. If the foods you eat raise your blood sugar at about the same rate as you burn it, you won't gain weight, and if the foods you eat raise your blood sugar more slowly than you burn it, the necessary energy will come from the liver and from body fat. You will lose weight.

Nondiabetics won't see their blood sugar rise like a diabetic's because everything works the way it's supposed to, so blood sugar is distributed for energy or fat storage automatically. You can't measure the impact of food by measuring your blood sugar. Your blood sugar won't go up like a diabetic's will, but eating foods that add glucose to your blood faster than you burn it or by adding more than you can burn, will still cause weight gain. The only way you can measure it is on your bathroom scale once a week. That's where it shows up.

In the following discussions of the various categories of food, pay close attention to my comments about how fast these foods will enter your bloodstream. This information will give you a fundamental key to understand which foods to eat to make lowering your blood sugar and losing weight easier than you ever dreamed it could be.

Grouping Food from a Diabetic's Perspective

This chapter provides a new look at grouping foods from a diabetic's perspective.

These groups are categorized based on what you now know are the key issues. *How fast* and *how much* each category of food will raise your blood sugar is of the utmost importance to all diabetics and anyone who wants to lose weight. Although this book has been written primarily for diabetics, everything I include with regard to healthier eating, weight loss, and activity applies equally to nondiabetics who want to lose weight and be healthier.

The Traditional Way of Describing Food Groups

One of the most important structural biology concepts that will help all diabetics understand and control blood sugars is that different foods have different molecular structures and therefore break down and enter your bloodstream as glucose at different speeds and different levels. This is vitally important to your understanding of why your blood sugars may sometimes seem unexplainable.

In the standard way of looking at food groups, if it's not a protein or fat, it's a carbohydrate. But this method confuses most of us and doesn't help you as a diabetic. The problem is that not all carbohydrates (carbs) act the same way or impact blood sugar, weight, or health the same way. For example, cauliflower is a carbohydrate and so is a sweet roll. Spaghetti's a carbohydrate and so is an apple. Bread is a carbohydrate and so is broccoli. Chocolate cake is a carbohydrate and so is cabbage. Pasta's a carbohydrate and so is a grapefruit. So how can you possibly talk about carbohydrates in general, because they are such a broad category and so different in their benefit and their impact on blood sugar and weight? No wonder people are so confused when they are told to eat fewer carbs. Does that mean less broccoli or less bread? Less spaghetti or fewer apples? This is not a good way to categorize foods and most people are understandably confused.

A New and Better Way of Grouping Foods for Diabetics Based on *How Much* and *How Fast* They Will Raise Blood Sugar

One of the prevailing problems I've encountered over the past 30 years as I talk to diabetics about foods is this: people know generally what fats are and can name some; they also know generally what proteins are and can name some. But carbohydrates are a different story. People are very confused about carbs.

Based on 30 years of testing, I've mentally divided carbohydrates into four groups based on how much and how fast they impact my blood sugar. Now I'm more formally introducing those groupings to help clarify America's "carb confusion."

The four discrete carbohydrate categories added to protein and fat compose the six food categories that will help you better understand what to eat and what not to eat. Here are the new six discrete groups of foods you need to memorize in order to better control your blood sugar and lose weight: sweet carbohydrates, starchy carbohydrates, fruit carbohydrates, veggie carbohydrates, proteins, and fats.

Each of these categories of foods plays a different role in blood sugar control and weight gain. Once you understand how each category of food reacts, your blood sugar control and weight control will improve dramatically. Here's your introduction to the categories.

Introduction to the Six Food Groups Based on Blood Sugar Impact

Sweet Carbohydrates

These molecules are very simple (mostly lone molecules or maybe two stuck together) and *easily dissolved and quick to enter your bloodstream*. Because they are the quickest of the food categories to enter your bloodstream and will cause the greatest rise in your blood sugar. Once again, remember that a rise in blood sugar means more insulin demand, which means more weight gain. This is not a new revelation except you will now see exactly how fast and how much this group will raise your blood sugar compared to other groups.

Starchy Carbohydrates

These foods have a slightly more complex molecular structure than sweet carbohydrates. Their molecules are stuck together in larger strings or branching chains which are a little harder to break apart and are just a little slower to enter your bloodstream than sweets, but will still have a fast and significant impact on blood sugar.

Fruit Carbohydrates

This category has quite a bit of variation in how fast and how much different fruits will increase blood sugar. Some fruit carbs act relatively slowly and cause moderate increases in blood sugar and some enter the bloodstream more quickly and will cause a moderate weight gain. The difference, of course, is in the food value and fiber that fruits have compared to sweets. Most fruits contain a variety of vitamins, minerals and fiber.

Veggie Carbohydrates

Veggie carbs are more complex than starchy carbohydrates and therefore slower to enter your bloodstream. In my testing I've learned that most veggie carbohydrates will raise your blood sugar less and more slowly than sweet carbs, starchy carbs, or fruit carbs. You'll see in the graphs that the impact of veggie carbs on your blood sugar is neither fast nor significant. There are a few exceptions of veggie carbs that act more like starchy carbs. Corn and potatoes are examples of this. Though they are considered vegetables, they act more like starchy carbs and will raise blood sugar significantly.

Proteins

The molecular structure of protein is more complex than the previous four food categories and slower to enter your bloodstream than sweet carbs, starchy carbs, and fruit carbs and about the same as most veggie carbs. So like veggie carbs, the rise in your blood sugar caused by proteins will be neither fast nor significant.

Fats

These are the slowest of all food categories to enter your bloodstream. The molecular structure of fat is complex, stable, and slow to show up in your bloodstream. To contrast it to sweet carbohydrates, which will show up in your bloodstream minutes after being eaten and will dramatically increase your blood sugar, fats alone have an almost negligible impact on blood sugar. Any impact fat does have on blood sugar is very slow and very small. Let me say this again. *Fat has very little impact on your blood sugar or on your weight. Fat alone will not make you fat.*

You'll note that I said "Fat *alone* will not make you fat." It's taken me 30 years to realize that neither fat nor protein, nor most veggie carbs alone will raise my blood sugar much and I've endured two major extreme low blood sugars requiring an ambulance trip to a hospital during this learning process. Once when I ate only roast beef and gave myself a normal dinner shot and once when I ate only shrimp and gave myself a normal dinner shot. Both times those foods hardly budged my blood sugar so my insulin shot was far too great.

What I've finally discovered through thousands of tests is only when proteins or fats are combined with starchy carbs—such as potatoes or bread with steak—or combined with sweet carbs—like a dessert after a steak dinner—do they cause a significant rise in blood sugar. That's why I said that fat *alone* does not make you fat.

I know this is counter to everything we've all been taught. It's counter to logic because, of course, if you put dietary fat in your mouth it must somehow transform into body fat and make its way to your waist or hips or your bottom. And besides, for 30 years the Federal Government through the USDA has been telling us to eat very little fat and eat lots of starchy carbs such as bread, cereal, rice, and pasta (six to 11 helpings a day). This information has become the core reference for hundreds of books and articles on healthy eating and Americans have gotten fatter and unhealthier every year since our government, the U.S. Department of Agriculture (USDA) first created this pyramid.

Some doctors and researchers who I will refer to later are leading the charge on this issue of fat not being your enemy, but it will be many years before the bloated federal bureaucracy works its ponderous way toward actively telling the American people that its food pyramid is now determined to be wrong and they no longer endorse it.

A Note about Calories

The final point I want to make before I discuss the specifics of the new six food groups and list the foods in each, is the difference in calories in each of these groups. I don't talk much about calories in this book because I'm dealing with what actually happens and what I can measure, not what theoretically should happen. But one researcher and author, Gary Taubes, who wrote *Good Calories, Bad Calories*, explains convincingly that "obesity is caused, not by the quantity of calories you eat but by the quality. Carbohydrates, particularly refined ones like white bread and pasta, raise insulin levels, promoting the storage of fat." I believe both he and Dr. Richard Bernstein, author of *The Diabetes Solution*, which I will refer to later, are on the right track to improve the health of Americans, diabetic or not.

More Detail on the Six Food Groups Used in This Book

This is not intended to be a comprehensive list of foods in each category but rather to give you a general understanding of which foods are in what groups and which will cause the greatest increases in your blood sugar and weight.

Sweet Carbohydrates

Here are examples of foods I include in this category: sugared soft drinks, cakes, pies, donuts, sweet rolls, ice cream, sherbets and sorbets, chocolates, caramels, a broad selection of desserts, and of course, candy.

We all know by now that too much sugar is the villain, right? Then what about all the *sugar-free* candies? Are they okay? Heck, they taste just like regular candy. But look closely at the label. You'll see that many of those items are sweetened with high-fructose corn syrup or with other sweeteners not much different from cane sugar except that they are more concentrated and make you fatter than plain cane sugar. So don't think you're doing yourself a favor by eating *sugar-free* candy. In terms of calories they are often the same and sometimes greater than sugared candy. Both regular candy and sugar-free candy are items you need to start minimizing dramatically. This is, of course, not new information but if you do all the other things I'll propose and still eat lots of candy, you're not going to make the progress you need or want.

Many of these sweet carbohydrates will show up as sugar in your bloodstream in two to three minutes. By drinking a soft drink, I can, for example, go from a low blood sugar of 50 mg/dl to 70 mg/dl in 90 seconds to 120 in three minutes. The simple sugars with no fat mixed in are the quickest to enter bloodstreams: sugared soft drinks, Skittles, jelly beans, and other candies that are pure sugar. Baked desserts such as cakes and pies usually have some fat in them, as do chocolate candy bars and ice cream. As you now know, fat enters your bloodstream more slowly, so when fat mixes with sweet carbohydrates in your stomach the combination is just slightly slower to enter your bloodstream than straight sweet carbohydrates, but the final impact is equal to or greater than that of pure sweets.

Take heart. In the next few chapters on actions to control blood sugar and lose weight, I'm not going to talk about cutting out desserts forever. But I will be talking about dramatically minimizing both the frequency and the quantity of desserts and sweets.

Okay. No big surprise so far. But here's a big one.

Starchy Carbohydrates

My next category of foods based on the speed of absorption and significance of the increase in blood sugar is starchy carbohydrates. Here are some examples of foods included in this category:

Waffles, pancakes, dry breakfast cereals, oatmeal, white and whole wheat bread, rolls, buns, muffins, tortillas, tortilla chips, potato chips, spaghetti, pasta, white rice, brown rice, crackers and similar foods.

Some vegetables belong with the starchy carbohydrates because of their impact on blood sugar: corn, potatoes, and baked beans are vegetables that act like starchy carbs, so I include them in the starchy carb category.

I don't eat many starchy carbs but when I do, I have to increase my insulin dosage to match the significant increase in my blood sugar that results. French fried potatoes are doubly bad because they're usually served fresh out of a Jacuzzi of hot grease. That combination of starchy carbs and fat (as you'll see later) is a bad combination, so I almost never order them, but I find myself nipping a few from my friends' plates because they do taste good. This falls under my philosophy of not needing to be perfect in your eating lifestyle.

Starchy Carbohydrates are certainly not as bad for you as sweet carbohydrates but they are significant contributors to blood sugar elevation and weight gain. One of the greatest favors you can do for yourself to lower your blood sugars and reduce your weight is to minimize your consumption of starchy carbohydrates as well as of sweet carbohydrates.

In consideration of how significant carbohydrates are to weight gain and blood sugar control, think about this. Almost all diabetic regimens require counting grams of carbohydrates or "counting carbs." This is the way to determine how much certain foods will raise your blood sugar and therefore how much insulin you will need. These regimens don't even advocate counting protein or fat. They don't count protein or fat because, by themselves, they have almost negligible impact on your blood sugar and consequently your weight. This fact alone speaks volumes about how important it is for you to control some carbohydrates (starchy carbs and sweet carbs) if you want to control your blood sugar and weight.

I'm not going to recommend cutting out starchy carbs but I will be suggesting that you should get as many of your carbs as possible from the veggie carb category and minimize the starchy carb category.

Now here's another surprise. Some fruits and especially fruit juices are going to also send your blood sugar up quite fast.

Fruit Carbohydrates

Many fruits will raise your blood sugar very fast. The fruits in this category are the following: pineapples, oranges, bananas, cherries, watermelons, peaches, pears, and strawberries. Cantaloupe, blueberries, and grapefruit do not raise my blood sugar as much as other fruits.

I don't mean to imply that fresh fruits are not good for diabetics. Fruits include many vitamins, minerals, and water-soluble fibers that are very important to general good health. But you do need to be aware that some fruits will cause significantly increased blood sugars and will contribute to weight gain. Fruits are not a free ride and have to be moderated by all diabetics to limit high blood sugars. Including some fresh fruit—but not too much—in a diabetic diet is a reasonable choice.

How about fruit juices? I've found that many fruit juices are problematic by causing very fast and very big blood sugar increases. In many cases a medium-size glass of *apple* juice or *orange* juice for breakfast will raise my blood sugar more than all the rest of my breakfast combined. And it gets into my bloodstream much faster than I can generally use it. So it gets stored in and on my body as fat.

An Associated Press article in the December 11, 2011 edition of the *Honolulu Star Advertiser* supports what I learned decades ago. The headline states, "Apple juice is far from nutritious, experts say." The article continues "…nutrition experts say apple juice's real danger is to waistlines and children's teeth. Apple juice has few natural nutrients, lots of calories, and in some cases, more sugar than soda. It trains a child to like very sweet things, displaces better beverages and foods, and adds to the obesity problem…".

In my personal experience, apple juice and orange juice both make my blood sugar skyrocket and require me to take more insulin than the fruits themselves require me to take. I don't drink pineapple juice but as sweet as it tastes, I expect it would act the same as apple and orange juice. Grapefruit juice does not raise my blood sugar as much or as fast as apple and orange but the increase is still notable. As a result of how much these juices impact my blood sugar, I dilute all the juices I drink to about 25 percent with 75 percent water or sparkling mineral water—in other words, one part juice to three parts water or Pelligrino (a sparkling mineral water).

Veggie Carbohydrates

Now we're getting to the really good stuff for lowering blood sugar and losing weight. Not only do these foods have lots of nutrients but they also enter your bloodstream more slowly than the previous three categories and cause an increase in blood sugar that's smaller than that caused by fruit carbs and way smaller than that of starchy or sweet carbs. This means that you can burn most of the calories from veggie carbohydrates before they get stored as glycogen or fat. For insulin-dependent diabetics it also means that your insulin injections or infusions can keep up with these foods and your blood sugar control will be much better.

These are the foods your mom told you to eat. She was right. They include most vegetables with the exception of the starchy ones I mentioned earlier. My favorite veggie carbohydrates are *asparagus, broccoli, tomatoes, cauliflower, artichokes, spinach, cabbage, carrots, peppers, mushrooms, beets, sauerkraut, and salad greens*. I pretty much eat all vegetables but draw the line at lima beans. "No thank you."

In the next few chapters you'll see that I speak often of maximizing protein and veggie carbohydrates, moderating fruit carbs, and minimizing sweet and starchy carbs.

So let's look at protein.

Protein

Protein has gone in and out of favor many times in the past 60 years. From the past 30 years of my blood sugar testing, I've learned that protein has very little effect on my blood sugar and a very noticeably positive effect on my muscle growth when I match protein with moderate strength training (chapter 11).

Because protein will cause neither a quick nor a significant rise in blood sugar, I freely eat large quantities of protein with almost no effect on my blood sugar or weight.

Examples of protein I eat often and freely are *salmon, halibut, crab, cod, trout, shrimp, and scallops.* I often include *chicken, turkey, and Cornish game hen* in my protein-eating patterns and will eat *beef, ham, and pork* as a change of pace. I don't eat veal because of the distressing way calves are confined for their whole lives to improve the taste and tenderness of veal.

My core protein food is Alaskan wild salmon. I eat salmon two or three times a week in the summer and once or twice a week in the winter. It's an almost perfect food. With very minimal impact on my blood sugar, it's absorbed slowly so it's burned as fast as it's absorbed and doesn't get stored as fat on my body. It's very high in protein and high in omega-3 fatty acids, which my secondary research indicates is an exceptionally good fat. Salmon is also a good source of vitamin D. All that and it tastes great too…as long as you don't overcook it.

Protein is a core food for muscle development. On my workout days, I'll often have an egg-white omelet either before or after working out—depending on how much aerobic exercise I'm planning on. I don't eat potatoes for breakfast anymore and rarely eat toast. I like egg whites not because the yolk is bad—it's only bad for you if you also eat toast or potatoes along with it— but because all of the protein is in the whites. An egg-white omelet usually contains about six egg whites as opposed to a typical egg omelet, which usually contains three full eggs. At seven grams of protein per egg white I get about 42 grams of protein in an egg-white omelet compared with about 21 grams of protein in a traditional egg omelet that includes the yolk.

Besides being a great source of protein, egg whites have almost zero impact on my blood sugar. Eating egg-white omelets is like drinking skim milk. If you get accustomed to skim milk, after a while whole milk tastes like cream—too rich. It's the same with egg-white omelets. There are, however, times when it okay to eat full eggs and times you should eat egg whites. You'll learn this later.

If you do decide to follow my advice and embark on a moderate, structured exercise program, you will need to consciously consume more protein or you'll see no results. On days when I exercise, I sometimes add a protein shake to my daily intake. I put in a small amount of frozen fruit, add two scoops of protein powder, some ice and the water, and blend it. That blended protein shake adds about 48 grams of protein to my daily intake. That combined with the 42 grams of protein from my egg-white omelet gets me almost half of my protein goal for workout days. If you're doing any strength training and want to see and feel results, you will need to consume more protein than a sedentary person.

I can attest from personal experience that consuming 150 to 200 grams of protein on the days of my workouts does noticeably enhance the results of my workouts. Though it's not something I can quantify precisely, it is something I can feel and see.

Fats *Fat Is Your Friend—But a Conditional Friend*
The impact of fats has been the biggest surprise to me over my years of testing. It took me a long time and thousands of blood tests to realize that fat alone has minimal impact on my blood sugar and almost no impact on weight gain. The reason it took me so long is that for years I almost always ate any fatty meats or butter with other foods, often with vegetables or starchy carbs. The latter, starchy carbs, as you will later see, is a bad combination with fat if eaten in the evening within two hours of going to bed. My evolving opinion about fats was confirmed in the tests that I have taken and graphed for this book.

Not many foods are all or predominantly fat, but here are a few of the foods that fall into the natural "fat" category: butter, olive oil, nuts, peanut butter, mayonnaise, and some salad dressings. Proteins that are high in fat include eggs (with the yolk), pork, bacon, prime rib, spareribs, many steaks (especially rib eye), hamburger, bratwurst, and mutton. Many of these foods are also loaded with protein, which adds to the positive benefit of them. Because protein and fat are often present in the same foods, it is difficult to test just fat but more practical to test protein and fat together.

Processed fats, while still in this category, are foods that I generally stay away from or at least minimize. Although I'm not an expert in this category, I am very apprehensive about the taste enhancers and chemicals added during the processing. Examples of the type of fats I avoid include margarine, fake butters, hot dogs (maybe I'll eat one a couple times a year at a football or baseball game), processed sandwich meats. Processed, precooked frozen dinners, which I haven't eaten for decades, are often in this category of processed fats.

Now that I've listed some of the high-fat foods, I'm going to attempt to persuade you in the balance of this chapter and in the next three chapters that natural fats (as opposed to processed fats) are not a problem and do not cause elevated blood sugars or weight gain as long as they're not eaten at or near the same time as starchy carbs or sweet carbs. You'll see graphs in chapter 6 illustrating that neither fatty proteins nor butter cause increases in blood sugar *unless* they are combined with starchy or sweet carbs. I'll also be explaining how my tests and experience measuring my own blood sugar concur with statements of some of the leading proponents of *higher-fat, low-carb diets.* I'll also be referring you to a number of medical researchers and doctors who argue convincingly that it's not fat that creates high cholesterol and high triglycerides levels, which are the big precursors of circulatory and heart problems, but it is foods that cause high blood glucose and call for high insulin production or injection.

As I said in the lead-in to this section, fats are not the villains they are made out to be. I know this is going to be a hard paradigm shift for Americans, because for years we've read over and over about losing weight with low-fat diets. We've read about low-fat this and low-fat that. Who argued? It seemed so reasonable. If you don't want to be fat then don't eat fat. It's simple, right? No... *wrong*.

Think about this for a minute—if eating fat makes people fat, one would think it would hold true for animals too. After all, enough similarities exist between mice and humans that mice are continually being tested by scientists to see how humans might react to the same food, medications, or environmental situations.

Let's just take cows, for example. Do cows eat fat? No, they're herbivores, grazers and foragers of grass and alfalfa. Grazing cows, like all other herbivores, naturally develop fat *without eating any fat*. But grazing took too long for cows to get fat enough.

Over the last 100 years in America, the beef industry has learned how to make cows "as fat as possible as fast as possible." How do they do it? They grow their cattle in feedlots on a diet of grain consisting primarily of corn. I'd call this corn-dominated grain "starchy carbohydrates for cows." They get much fatter much faster than cows grazing on the prairies. How often have you heard or read the term "pure corn-fed beef." Corn-dominated feed makes cows fat quickly and gives beef a juicier, fattier texture—and likely a better taste. This is great for the beef industry and for all of us who like a tasty, juicy steak once in a while, but is this what you want for yourself—to get *as fat as possible as fast as possible*? Cows get this way almost exclusively on corn-dominated rations (starchy carbs for cows).

If you are one of those rare Americans who are underweight and want to gain weight fast this is how to do it. Eat lots of starchy carbohydrates. Throw in lots of processed foods often loaded with starchy carbs and finish off each meal with sweet carbohydrates. But don't waste your time trying to gain weight by eating a lot of natural fats because it's not going to happen. In the words of Dr. Rob Bennedetti, the chair of the Medical Division of Rockwood Clinic in Spokane, "Nobody ever got fat by eating too many avocados." I don't mean to imply that Dr. Bennedetti agrees with everything I say about fat but the quote was too good to pass up.

I puzzled for years about the fact that fatty foods for breakfast (bacon or sausage and eggs) sometimes raised my blood sugar and insulin demand and sometimes they didn't. It took me at least 20 years of testing my blood to figure out what was happening. As long as I didn't eat starchy carbs like toast, muffins, potatoes, or pancakes with the bacon, eggs, or sausage then the fat would have almost no impact on my blood sugar but if I had any starchy carbs with the bacon, eggs, or sausage, my blood sugar would go up significantly. By the end of the next chapter you'll have an understanding of the relationship between fat and starchy carbs that will dramatically improve your health.

To further support my message that dietary fat does not make you fat and dietary cholesterol does not add to blood cholesterol, I've added this paragraph from an article that appeared in the *New York Times* three days before this book was scheduled to go to press.

> "The Dietary Guidelines Advisory Committee, which convenes every five years, followed the lead of other major health groups like the American Heart Association that in recent years have backed away from dietary cholesterol restrictions and urged people to cut back on added sugars."

New York Times
February 19, 2015

Chapter 6

Visual Impact of Foods on Blood Sugar and Weight

Testing Foods Impact on Blood Sugar— 60,000 Tests and Counting

It's taken me 30 years, and to the best of my calculations over 60,000 blood sugar tests, to learn what you will learn in these next three chapters about food.

Though I'm in my 50th year with diabetes, self-testing has been available for a little more than 30 years. In the years before self-testing the only way I could get a blood sugar measurement was to set an appointment with my doctor who would give me a lab request. I then had to go to a lab to have a blood sample taken. The lab would send it out to an analytical lab and get the result back in three days. They would then call my doctor who would have a staff person call me and tell me what my blood sugar had been three or four days prior. Because of that cumbersome process, I had my blood sugar tested only three or four times a year.

I now self-test when I wake up each morning, before each meal, often between meals and before I go to bed each night. I also test before physical activities and many times after these activities as well as any other time I think my blood sugar needs adjusting. As a result of all these tests I've learned how hundreds of different foods will impact my blood sugar and weight. I've learned not only how *much* different foods will raise my blood but also how *fast* those foods will raise my blood sugar.

For Type 1 diabetics, both *how much* and *how fast* certain foods will make your blood sugar go up are very important. Knowing those two factors and being able to predict the action of certain foods will help immensely in your ability to anticipate and control your blood sugar levels with injected or infused insulin.

For Type 2 diabetics, borderline diabetics, pre-diabetics, and anyone who wants to lose weight, *how much* and *how fast* different foods raise your blood sugar is also important. *How much* is important because the more a food raises your blood sugar, the more that food will demand more effort from your pancreas and require it to try to produce more insulin or require you to inject more insulin. More insulin (whether you inject it or your pancreas produces it) means more weight gain. So when you see on the graphs in this chapter showing certain foods that will significantly raise your blood sugar. Remember that means those foods will also contribute to significant weight gain. How *fast* foods raise blood sugar is also very important for anyone who wants to lose weight or avoid gaining weight. If certain foods raise your blood sugar faster than you can burn that sugar, it will be stored in your liver or in fat cells around your body. That's bad. That means weight gain. But if certain foods raise your blood sugar at about the same speed or slower than you burn those calories, then those calories will be used before they are stored. That's good. That means weight stability or weight loss.

This is a good point to state that I can personally measure only the impact of foods on blood sugar and weight. I can't make any judgments from my empirical testing with regard to the impact of vitamins, minerals or other ingredients that don't relate to blood sugar.

While this book is written primarily for people with diabetes, it also applies directly to all the two thirds of American adults who the Center for Disease Control says are overweight or obese.

My Methodology for Testing Foods (and Drinks)

Over the past 30 years of eating then testing my blood sugar and trying to match my insulin injections with foods I've eaten, I've learned a lot about which foods cause the greatest blood sugar increases and weight gain and which cause the least blood sugar increases and weight gain. I've continually adjusted my diet to respond to that information.

But for the purposes of this book I've conducted very specific tests on blood sugar impact and therefore weight gain impact of multiple foods in all of the six food groups. I've graphed each of those tests to clearly show what foods you should minimize to avoid large increases in blood sugar and therefore weight gain and what foods you can maximize with little rise in blood sugar and therefore weight loss. The results will surprise you.

The purpose of the graphs I present in this chapter is to provide visual representations of what I've learned from the 60,000 blood tests I given myself over the past 35 years. These graphs will make it easier for the readers to visualize and remember what food groups and foods within the groups will elevate blood sugars and add weight and what food groups and foods will not.

As a Type 1 diabetic, my body produces no insulin at all but whatever food or combinations of foods I eat are converted to glucose in my blood just as it is for everyone, diabetic or not. But if I don't give myself a shot of insulin when I eat that food, my blood sugar will just keep on rising until I do give myself a shot. That's precisely how I can measure the blood sugar impact and therefore fat gain impact of individual foods and combinations of foods and graph those results.

In order to make these graphs as accurate a representation as I could, I followed the same protocol for each of the food tests. I first made sure my blood sugar was stable—that it was not going up or down. To assure that stability, most of my tests were done in the morning when I hadn't eaten anything for at least 10 hours. I've adjusted my insulin pump base rate to compensate for the dawn syndrome (explained later). That adjustment means that if I ate nothing after I woke up my blood sugar would remain stable. To confirm that my blood sugar was stable, I would test two or three times before I ate or drank the foods or drinks to be tested.

Once I was sure my blood sugar was stable, I would then consume the test food or drink. The next step was to set my smart phone to alert me every ten minutes for 90 minutes. I made a special effort to burn energy consistently during the tests so the results wouldn't be skewed even slightly by more or less activity. I usually read the paper, a magazine, or a book during the tests. While reading I was nine steps away from the counter upon which my testers and the charts I recorded were placed. That meant 18 steps back and forth every ten minutes for each test. Counting duplicate tests to confirm, on average I stuck my fingers and tested about 12-15 times within every 90 minute period.

At the end of 90 minutes I took an appropriate shot of insulin which—in about an hour—brought my blood sugar back to a normal range. But those 90 minutes before I took that insulin shot tell a story. They tell a story that can improve the lives of millions of Americans; a story that can help millions of Type 2 diabetics lower their blood sugars and lose weight; a story that can prevent millions of Americans from ever getting diabetes; and a story that can help Type 1 diabetics achieve better control of their blood sugars.

The final point I need to make in describing my methodology is that whatever stable point my blood was when I started, I indexed it to 100. What that means is if I established that my starting blood sugar was say 112 and stable, then my index was minus 12. That means I subtracted 12 points from my starting level and 12 points from every measurement for the full 90 minutes. And if for example my starting point was 84, I added 16 points to my starting level and 16 to each test for the full 90 minutes. That process gives every test the same starting point and will show slopes, peaks, and areas that can be accurately compared.

With that explanation, I still want to emphasize that these tests are to illustrate what I have learned from tens of thousands of previous tests. The graphs themselves would not be sufficient evidence of my conclusions. But because they coincide with my results from the 60,000 previous tests, I feel very comfortable with the validity of these graphs.

The findings are dramatic and likely different from what you've read or been told about food. The conclusions will change your eating lifestyle, your health and your enjoyment of life. It's not about a short term diet but rather about eating in a healthy way that you will enjoy for the rest of your life—eating *smaller* portions of the foods which maximize your blood sugars and contribute to weight gain and eating *larger* portions of the foods will have minimal effect on blood sugars and which will contribute to weight loss.

Will the foods I've graphed have the same impact on everyone else as they have had on me?

The answer is "Not exactly". Different size people have different volumes of blood circulating through their body so the impact will vary based on the volume of blood in a person's body. A small female may have as little as five pints of blood circulating in her body but a large male could have 10 pints or more circulating in his body. If a very small female, for example, ate the same foods and same size portions of foods I did, the impact on her blood sugar and weight would be proportionally greater than the impact on my blood sugar and weight. If a 260 pound male (I weight between 185 and 190) ate the same foods and portion sizes I did, the impact on his blood sugar and weight would be proportionally less than the impact on my blood sugar and weight.

While the impact of my tests won't be exactly the same for everyone, the slopes, the peaks, and the shaded area of the graphs will still give an valid comparison of foods to each other. If food "A" causes my blood sugar to rise *faster* than food "B", there is no reason it would not do the same for you. If food "C" causes my blood sugar to rise more than food "D" it will do the same for you.

The slower a food or drink cause my blood sugar to rise—again, the *slope*— the less likely it will be stored as fat because I will be burning more of that food as energy before it gets a chance to be stored and the same will hold for you.

The higher the *peak* of the graph means that food or combination of foods had a greater impact on my blood sugar than a food or drink with a lower peak. The same will hold true for you.

Finally the greater the *shaded area* beneath the slope line, the more impact that food had on my weight and the more impact that food (or drink) will have on your weight.

While the absolute numbers may vary based on the weight and size of an individual, the relative impact of the foods or drinks tested will be valid. That's okay because the purpose is for you to see how different foods compare with one another in terms of blood sugar and weight gain.

In this book I'm not going to tell you to eat this many grams of this food or that many ounces of that food or this many calories per meal. I don't count calories or grams. Those ideas and methods haven't worked well for Americans. While authors continually promote counting calories, Americans keep getting fatter and fatter. While being aware of calories is somewhat important what's more important is how much any food raises blood sugar. As you review the charts you'll see that 200 calories of protein, vegetables, and—yes—even fat alone will raise your blood sugar a lot less and contribute less to your weight gain than 200 calories of sweet or starchy carbs. My purpose is to show you visuals of how each of these six food categories act and how foods within these categories act.

I'm betting that after you read this book, you'll be showing people at work, at the office or at any social gatherings what the slopes of different foods are like by using your hands to imitate those slopes. These graphs will find a secure place in your memory and always be there. You'll always remember what foods will contribute more to blood sugar and weight gain and what foods will contribute less to blood sugar and therefore to weight loss.

Interpreting the Graphs—A Review

The **slopes** of the graphs tell a Type 1 and insulin dependent Type 2 diabetic how *fast* each food or combination of foods will increase blood sugar and therefore how much insulin is required. The **peaks** of the graphs tell all diabetics how *much* each food or combination of foods will increase their blood sugars. And the **shaded area** under the slope line gives a general indication of the total weight gain each food or combination of foods contributes to diabetics and non-diabetics alike.

Most people can only get feedback on the impact of foods only *once or twice a week* or *once or twice a month* when they step on scale. They can only speculate on which of the foods they ate contributed to weight gain or loss. I get feedback six or more times *a day* and this is the information I will share with you.

During Anchorage's Olympic Bids, I recall the International Olympic Committee member from China, He Zhenlaiang—after his visit to Anchorage—making a comment to me that I have never forgotten. We were riding together on the way back to the airport after his visit to Anchorage. He turned to me and said, "Mr. Chairman, I've heard you speak at many meetings around the world but I've forgotten much of what you said. When I saw your visual presentations, I remembered. Now that I've visited your city, I understand."

I think the visual presentations of the graphs will help you remember. But when you start seeing the resulting improved blood sugars and weight loss, *you'll understand.*

A Note on the Graphs

As you review these graphs, you'll see that foods typical to breakfasts are measured and graphed more often than other meals. There are two reasons I've done this. First, breakfast is a meal that people tend to eat the same or similar things most mornings so getting into a better pattern of eating is easier. Second, there seems to be more misinformation about healthy breakfast foods than other meals. But because I've been testing for so long and so frequently, I know that whatever the meal, breakfast, lunch, dinner, or snacks; all of the foods within the food groups act similarly.

The final note before you get into the graphs is that you will see some graphs have slight dips between 40 and 70 minutes. This happens because my pump is putting a tiny maintenance amount of insulin into my body continuously. It's called the basal rate. Not unlike the small amount of glycogen put into the body by the liver. What that small decrease reflects is my body using a small amount of that glucose just walking up to my tester and back to my seat. My body would use roughly the same amount for all foods tested but in some cases glucose is going in so fast that a slight dip doesn't show. This effect does not significantly change the results.

Key to Graphs

The horizontal axis represents the time in minutes that I measured my change in blood sugar.

The vertical axis represents the rise in my blood sugar measured in milligrams per deciliter (mg/dl). The starting point is always indexed to 100.

The Slope (the angled line) represents speed of the rise in blood sugar; the steeper the slope, the faster the rise in blood sugar.

The shaded area is a general representation of the total contribution to weight gain. That contribution will be offset somewhat by activity, exercise, and just day-to-day living. The larger the gray area the less likely that all the glucose will be needed and used for energy and the more likely some of that glucose will be stored as fat.

What to Look for in the Graphs

Now let's take a first look at how different foods impact blood sugar and weight. By the time you finish reviewing these graphs you'll have a strong visual memory of which foods you must minimize to lower blood sugar and lose weight and which foods you can maximize with no impact on weight gain. By understanding and applying the information in these graphs Type 1 diabetics will have better control their blood sugar, Type 2 diabetics will lower their blood sugar and lose weight, and prediabetics or borderline diabetics will avoid ever getting diabetes.

As you look at these graphs, it's most important that you go back and forth and see how the six different groups compare with one another. No one—including me—can ever know how much *every* food we'll ever eat will contribute to blood sugar and weight but you don't have to. Your primary goal should be to understand which food groups are the biggest contributors to high blood sugar and weight gain and which are not. Your secondary goal should be which foods groups when combined with others will have little impact on weight and which food groups when combined with others will have maximum impact on blood sugar and weight. The details of these good and bad combinations will be covered in more detail in the next chapter.

Sweet Carbohydrates

I'm going to start with sweet carbs. We all know they make your blood sugar go up and contribute substantially to weight gain. No surprise here. But these graphs will give readers perspective on how much and how fast this happens. It also gives a point of reference for the rest of the food categories.

Here's a review of foods in this category.

Regular, sweetened (non-diet) soft drinks, candy bars, cakes, pies, donuts, sweet rolls, sweet toppings for ice creams, chocolates, caramels, other sweetened candies, sweet desserts. We all know by now that too much sugar is a villain. Then what about all the *sugar-free* candies? Are they okay? Heck, they taste just like regular candy. But look closely at the label. You'll see that many of those items are sweetened with high fructose corn syrup or with other sweeteners like sucrose, not much different than cane sugars but a little more concentrated and therefore worse for you. So don't think you're doing yourself a favor by eating *sugar-free* candy. It only means the manufacturers use concentrated sweeteners other than sugar. Both regular candy and sugar-free candy are items that you need to start minimizing or eliminating. This is, of course, not new information but if you do all the other things I'll propose and still eat lots of candy, you're not going to make the progress you need or want.

Cherry Danish

This is my all-time record holder for increasing my blood sugar. It went from 100 to 458 in 90 minutes. This caused a net blood sugar rise of 358 mg/dl in 90 minutes. This is a huge rise and a great contributor to weight.

   Notice that the net blood sugar rise is 100 points less than my final blood sugar on the graph. The reason is, of course, that all my blood sugars started or were indexed to 100, which is within the generally accepted normal levels, so the starting point must subtracted from the finishing blood sugar to get the net rise.

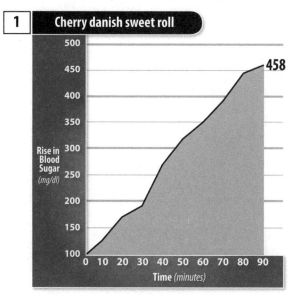

Net blood sugar rise – 358*

Apple Pie

This is another very big rise in blood sugar. In my experience this blood sugar rise is typical of most pies. Whether you cut out desserts like this, eat them less frequently or dramatically reduce portion size will be up to you. The important thing right now is to lock this visual in your mind. Most pies and cakes will act similarly to this. Though I only eat pie or cake maybe a dozen times a year, their combination of sweet carbs and starchy carbs have always caused the biggest rises in my blood sugars. I can cover it with a huge infusion of insulin that is often larger than the infusion for the complete meal preceding it. That means the pie or cake would raise my blood sugar more and make me fatter than all the rest of the food on my plate combined.

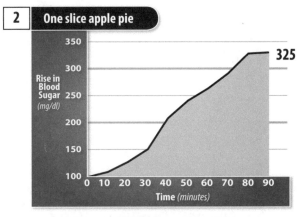

Net blood sugar rise – 225

Chocolate Covered Donut

Here's another food that has an impact even greater than most would expect. Donuts are a very common breakfast habit for many people. If you eat a donut or a sweet roll for breakfast and wonder why you're gaining weight, compare this graph to other breakfast choices shown in later graphs.

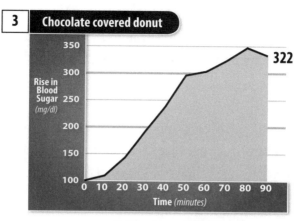

Net blood sugar rise – 222

Hershey Bar

I've included a Hershey Bar graph because it such a common candy bar and people can relate to it. I also use a Hershey Bar in future chapters to illustrate how much making a small change in habits can mean over a year. Both the slope and the impact are less than the first three graphs but still significant. A Hershey Bar has 210 calories. Compare this graph to eggs (graphs 42 and 43). Three large eggs also have 210

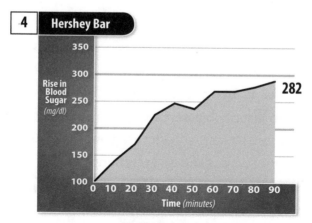

Net blood sugar rise – 182

calories, exactly the same as a Hershey Bar but look at how much less three eggs contribute to blood sugar and weight than a Hershey bar does. Calories are only pertinent if one is comparing like foods.

Coke

I've included a graph of eight ounces of Coca Cola (most Coke bottles or cans are 12 ounces) because I wanted to provide a point of comparison with fruit juices that I've graphed in the fruit carbs' group.

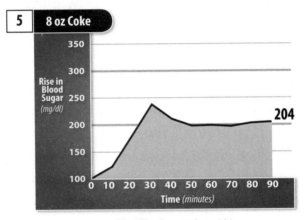

Net blood sugar rise – 104

Ice Cream or Sorbet

I'm sorry to report that ice cream in its various forms is a big problem for blood sugar elevation and weight gain. As you'll find out in the next chapter, the combination of sweet carbs and fat is not good. You'll also understand why that combination should be avoided late in the evening. If you really love ice cream—doesn't everyone—and can't do without it, eat it earlier in the day and do everything you can to minimize it. For a smaller impact—as well as a great taste, I eat Haagen Dazs Zesty Lemon Sorbet. It has sweet carbs but no fat as far as I can tell by my blood sugar reaction; notice that my blood sugar starts to drop after about 40 minutes. For this test, I ate about a half-pint which is huge for me. When I do eat it, I typically eat just a couple of tablespoons at a time so a pint may last me a month. But it is very refreshing.

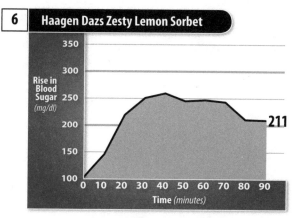

Net blood sugar rise – 111

Conclusions Regarding the Sweet Carbohydrates Group

First of all there are no surprises here. We all know sweets are a big contributor to high blood sugars and significant weight gain. But it's important that sweet carbohydrates are included here so you can compare their reaction to the other five categories.

It's also important to know that if you're a Type 1 or insulin dependent Type 2 diabetic it will be very hard for your injected or infused insulin to keep up with those quick increases in blood sugar. You will have spikes in your blood sugars.

Starchy Carbohydrates

My next category of foods based on the speed of absorption and total impact on blood sugar and weight is starchy carbohydrates. Here are some examples of foods I include in this category: waffles, pancakes, breakfast cereals—including oatmeal—, breads, rolls, buns, muffins, tortillas, tortilla chips, potato chips, spaghetti, pasta, crackers and other wheat products. I categorize some vegetables as starchy carbohydrates because of the speed and amount of blood sugar increases they cause. In other words they act like starchy carbs in terms of weight gain but are generally considered vegetables. Corn and potatoes are in this group. When I eat them I have to adjust my insulin dosage for significant increases in my blood sugar as a result.

In looking at this group of graphs for the first time it will still be hard for you to put them in perspective but after completely reviewing all the graphs, you'll want to go back and forth and compare the impacts of each group. This group, I believe will be one of the biggest surprises to most people.

Spaghetti

This graph shows the impact of a starchy carbohydrate if eaten without sauce, butter or other flavorings. Normally it would not be eaten this way but my purpose in this graph is to illustrate the blood sugar and weight gain impact of just starchy carbs. Note how much slower blood sugar goes up when fat (butter) is added to the spaghetti. This gives you more time to burn the glucose before it is stored.

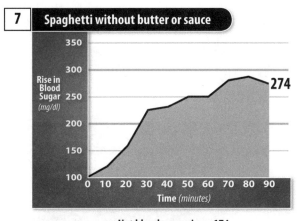

Net blood sugar rise – 174

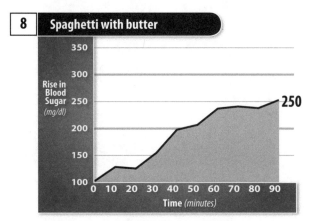

Net blood sugar rise – 150

Potatoes

Note how much slower potatoes with butter and sour cream enter the blood stream. This gives you a better chance to burn the glucose before it gets stored. We would all be better off if we ate half as much potato with twice as much butter and sour cream.

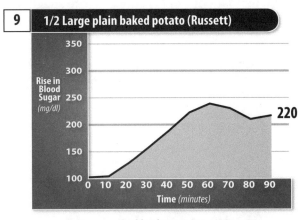

Net blood sugar rise – 120

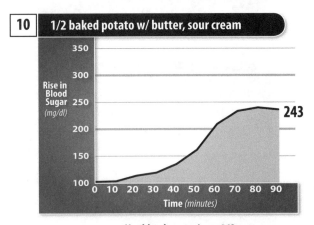

Net blood sugar rise – 143

Oatmeal

Oatmeal is widely considered to be a very healthy breakfast and you will see that it is similar to the other cereals that I've graphed with regard to blood sugar and weight contribution. However, as you continue with this chapter, you will see that other choices will be better for blood sugar control and weight loss.

Remember what I said earlier in this chapter; I can't make any judgments from my empirical testing with regard to the impact of vitamins, minerals or other ingredients that don't relate to blood sugar.

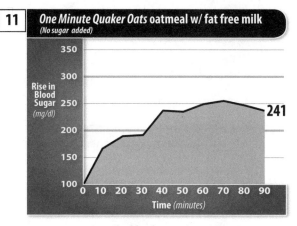

Net blood sugar rise – 141

Cereal

Most cereals seem to identify about the same range of calories in their nutrition facts—usually between 100 and 130 but as you will see later

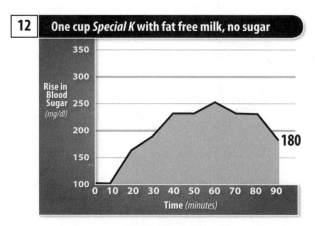

Net blood sugar rise – 80

13 | **One cup *Cheerios* with fat free milk, no sugar**

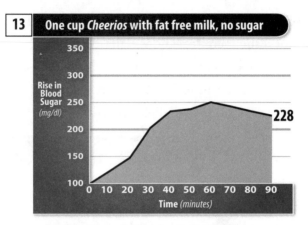

228

Net blood sugar rise – 128

14 | **One cup *Total* with fat free milk, 1 tsp sugar**

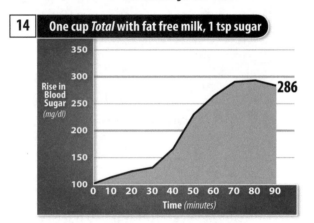

286

Net blood sugar rise – 186

15 | **One cup Total and whole milk** *(No sugar added)*

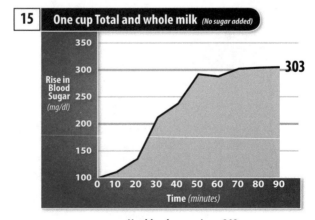

303

Net blood sugar rise – 203

calories and blood sugar, and calories and weight gain are not always related. Some foods with fewer calories may have more impact on blood sugar and weight gain than other foods with more calories. When you compare these cereal graphs with graphs of two eggs which have about 140 calories, you'll begin to understand that statement. I don't eat much cereal because of the big impact on my blood sugar and weight but I chose Total to test because it looked the healthiest from the box information. The results of these tests are quite consistent with my general experience with many different cereals until I stopped eating them about 15 years ago.

Granola

Terry and David's Double Nut Granola

I don't recall ever eating granola as a breakfast cereal before this test so I didn't know what to expect. But, like many Americans I always associated granola with good health so I was very surprised by the results of my testing.

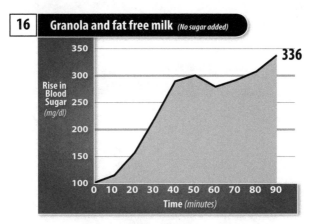

Net blood sugar rise – 236

Bagels

Bagels seem to be a food that people who are health conscious eat. I've often heard folks say with a certain modicum of self-pride, "I usually just have a bagel and cream cheese for breakfast." With that statement in mind, I tested, not with a full bagel, but with one-half bagel with cream cheese and then a bagel without cream cheese or butter. If this is what a half bagel does, think about the impact of a full bagel. You'd be getting into cherry Danish territory. On graph 18, the

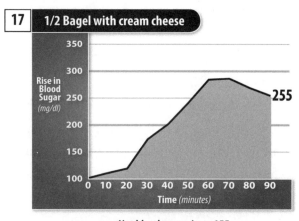

Net blood sugar rise – 155

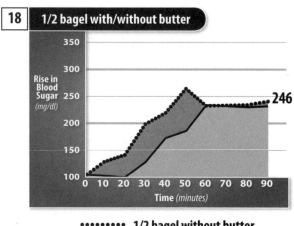

•••••••• 1/2 bagel without butter
———— 1/2 bagel with butter

light gray area is a bagel with butter. The dark gray added to the light gray is a bagel without butter. The butter slows down the entry of glucose into the blood stream and gives you more opportunity to burn the glucose before it gets stored.

Wheat Toast

When I do eat toast, which is not often any more, I choose wheat toast. From everything I've read wheat toast is better than white toast. I can't measure that but as I have with cereal, I've gradually reduced the

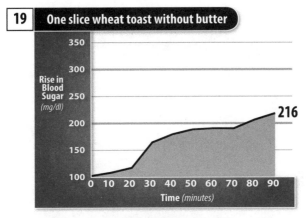

Net blood sugar rise – 116

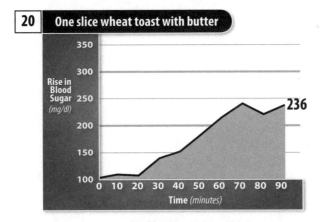

Net blood sugar rise – 136

number of bread products that I eat because of their discouragingly high increases in my blood sugar and therefore weight from them.

Gluten Free Toast

Gluten free toast is not something I'm familiar with nor have I eaten prior to the tests graphed below so I can't say that the few tests I took are absolute certainties but the corn starch and tapioca starch in gluten free bread appear to have a slightly smaller impact on my blood sugar than the wheat in other breads.

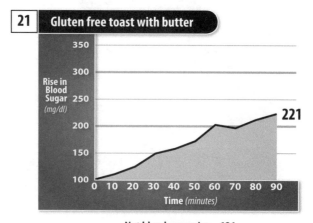

Net blood sugar rise – 121

Conclusions Regarding the Starchy Carbohydrate Group

It's been my experience as a result of thousands of blood sugar tests that starchy carbs will raise my blood sugar almost as much as sweet carbs. I'm not suggesting that sweet carbs and starchy carbs are equivalent in terms of general health. I'm confident that starchy carbs are probably the better of the two, but if you want to lower blood sugars, control blood sugar swings, and lose weight, dramatically reducing starchy carbs is absolutely necessary.

A Note on Healthy Active Children

This is a good point to remind readers that the eating suggestions I make here are geared toward adults and not young, active, growing children. If children are overweight or obese then they would do well by following the advice in my eating recommendations, but if they're of normal weight, active, and growing I'm not making these recommendations for them especially with regard to starchy carbs. Children who are going out to play for three or four hours after breakfast will do fine with cereal and toast but if they're going to sit in a classroom or in front of a computer or television they should cut back somewhat on starchy carbs for breakfast.

Once you see the graphs of how the next four categories of foods act you'll begin to be able to visually compare how much starchy carbs and sweet carbs contribute to high blood sugar and weight gain.

Fruit Carbohydrates

The foods in this category are quite obvious. Almost everyone knows what fruits are: apples, oranges, pineapples, oranges, bananas, watermelons, peaches, pears, berries, etc.

Fruit carbs are certainly better than sweet carbs and starchy carbs in terms of blood sugar and weight control. They also are known to provide more healthful nutrients than the first two categories. But are they a free ride? Can you eat as much fruit as you wish without significant blood sugar increases and weight gain? I'll start with the fruits that have the highest impact on blood sugar and weight gain and move to fruits with lower impact on blood sugar and weight.

Bananas

Bananas have the highest impact on my blood sugar of the fruits that I eat. I stopped eating pineapples many years ago because they raised my blood sugar so much. That, I think, is obvious to most people because of the extraordinary sweetness of that fruit. But bananas don't have that sweet taste so their impact would be hard for someone to tell just based on taste. In the graph below, you'll see the impact of a banana on blood sugar and contribution to weight gain is big. You'll also notice a drop at about 50 minutes which I explained just prior to the graph section. Also consider for a moment adding a banana to the cereal graphs that you just saw. That combination creates a big, big impact on blood sugar and substantial contribution to weight gain.

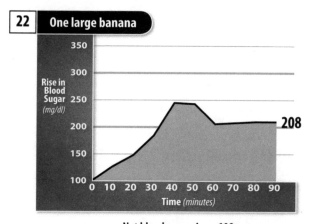

Net blood sugar rise – 108

Queen Anne Cherries

I eat a small to moderate amount of cherries—usually Queen Anne or Bing Cherries. I have, over the years, brought the quantity I eat down because of their fairly high impact on my blood sugar. Be careful about eating too many cherries.

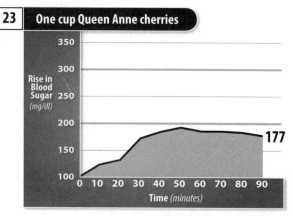

Net blood sugar rise – 77

Oranges

Oranges are in the middle of fruits in terms of fruits in terms of blood sugar control and weight contribution. Not too bad but not as good as ones to come. I'm a fan of quartering oranges and eating as much of the fiber (what your mom called roughage) as I can.

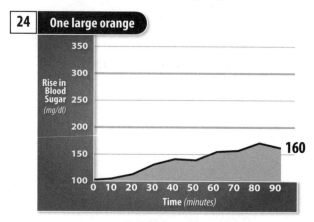

Net blood sugar rise – 60

Blackberries

Blackberries have about the same impact as oranges. They're not too bad in terms of blood sugar impact but you still won't want to splurge on them.

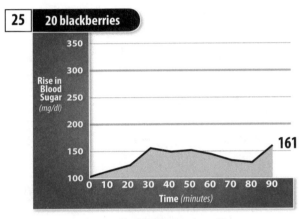

Net blood sugar rise – 61

Apples

Apples are pretty darn good; not too much impact on blood sugar or weight and not much likelihood of over indulging by eating two or three apples.

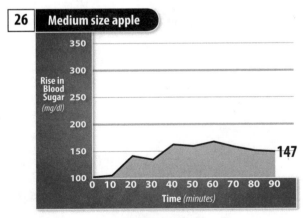

Net blood sugar rise – 47

Blueberries

Not only will blueberries have little influence on your blood sugar and weight but everything I've read praises them for all their healthy ingredients.

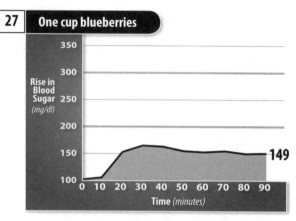

27 One cup blueberries

149

Net blood sugar rise – 49

Cantaloupe

Cantaloupe in season is one of my favorite breakfast fruits. My helpings are usually pretty big and the impact on my blood sugar and weight is very small. This is a fruit that because of its sweet taste, I expected to have a greater impact on my blood sugar than it does.

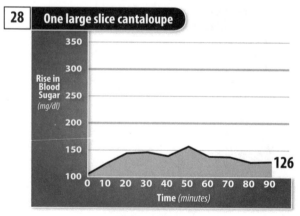

28 One large slice cantaloupe

126

Net blood sugar rise – 26

Grapefruit

This graph disagrees with some things I've read about grapefruit but my 30 year experience with grapefruit is consistent with what this graph shows. By the way I haven't put sugar on anything since I got diabetes and I don't miss it. I don't use artificial sweeteners on or in anything either because I believe that contributes to maintaining a taste and desire for sweeter things.

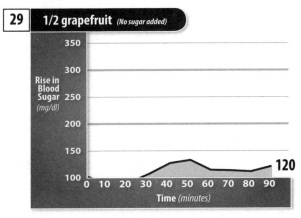

Net blood sugar rise – 20

Conclusions Regarding the
Fruit Carbohydrate Group

Despite the vitamins, minerals and general health benefits fruits offer they are not a free ride. In other words they will contribute moderately to increased blood sugar and weight gain. A Type 1 diabetic needs to be attentive to the slopes of the graphs and a Type 2 diabetic who is trying to lower blood sugars and anyone trying to lose weight needs to be moderate in their consumption of fruits—especially pineapples, bananas, and cherries, and blackberries.

Fruit Juices

Still within my category of fruit carbohydrates are fruit juices. Following are graphs for three of the most common juices: apple juice, orange juice, and grapefruit juice. I've also tested and graphed my "go to juice" V-8 which will give an interesting point of reference. Compare the graphs of these juices to an 8 oz. glass of Coke that's a few pages back in the sweet carbs group.

In all of the fruit juice graphs, it's important to note how fast the juices increase blood sugar. Because of these fast increases, pay special attention to the volume of the gray area created by the fruit juices as compared to V-8 juice which has a significantly smaller gray shaded area because of its slower blood sugar increase. It therefore has a much smaller contribution to weight gain. This is a very important concept to grasp. Even if the end point is the same, the slower the rise, the greater the opportunity to burn glucose before it is stored and therefore the less the contribution to weight gain.

Apple Juice

Note that the net blood sugar increase from apple juice is 133 mg/dl. That approaches three times the 47 mg/dl blood sugar increase of a medium-size apple (graph 26). But even more important than that, note the huge difference in the volume of the shaded area of the apple juice compared to an apple. This is a dramatic visualization of the huge contribution to weight increase of the juice compared to the fruit.

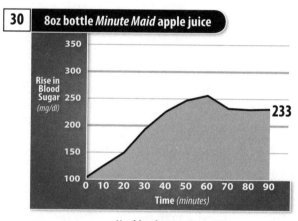

Net blood sugar rise – 133

Orange Juice

Orange juice provides a similar comparison though not as dramatic as apple juice. The net rise in blood sugar caused by orange juice is 121 mg/dl compared to 60 for a large orange. Once again though, because the orange juice increases blood sugar so much faster, the shaded area representing the juice's contribution to weight gain is significantly larger than the orange itself.

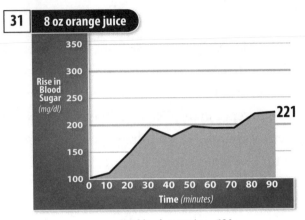

31   **8 oz orange juice**

Net blood sugar rise – 121

Grapefruit Juice

Now compare grapefruit juice to ½ grapefruit (graph 29). Not only does the juice cause a much bigger rise than the grapefruit itself but because it causes such a fast rise, it goes into your blood stream faster than you can use it and much of the glucose it causes—just like apple juice and orange juice—will end up being stored. This comparison also shows the net blood sugar rise for ½ grapefruit of 20 mg/dl

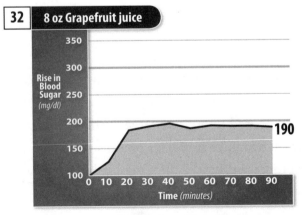

32   **8 oz Grapefruit juice**

Net blood sugar rise – 90

144

compared to a net rise of the juice of 90. Now some will argue that I should have compared a full grapefruit to 8 oz. of juice. They may be right but my goal here is to compare typical portions. I don't ever recall seeing anyone eating two grapefruit halves in a restaurant but I often see folks drinking 8 oz. or more of whatever juice they ordered. Even if I were to double the grapefruit portion, it would still be less than ½ of the increase in blood sugar of the juice.

V-8 Juice

This graph is a good illustration of the value of foods or liquids that cause slower rises in blood sugar. In this case the V-8 juice reaches the same quite-high level that the other juices do but it reaches that level much slower. Over a 90 minute period as shown in these graphs, the very slow rise in glucose means less of the glucose created by V-8 juice will be stored since you'll be burning it as it enters. You won't be able to burn the glucose from the other juices as fast as they go in so the excess glucose will be stored as fat.

I can rarely get V-8 in restaurants but it is the juice of choice for me at home. For the past few years I've been diluting about a third of

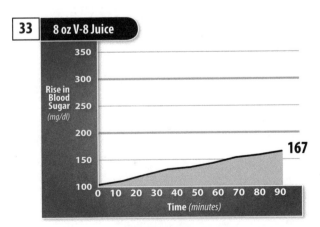

Net blood sugar rise – 67

a large glass of V-8 juice with two thirds of a glass of Pellegrino Sparkling Mineral Water. It's now not only my favorite breakfast drink but also a very refreshing mid-day drink.

Conclusions Regarding Fruit Juices

Diluting your morning fruit juice is one of the easiest actions you can take. The impact on your blood sugar and weight will, of course, depend on how much juice you drink now. Go back and compare apple juice and orange juice to the Coke (graph 5). While the nutritional value of the juices is greater than a Coke so is the impact on your blood sugar and weight.

As I've mentioned my preference is to dilute my juice with Pellegrino Sparkling Mineral Water. But whether you dilute your juice with mineral water or tap water, you'll soon find the diluted juice becoming an easy pattern that will become a habit in no time. It's one of those small actions that will make a big difference over time.

Vegetable Carbohydrates

Now we're getting into the really good stuff. Your mother was right; eat your vegetables. She probably told you they would make you healthy but what she didn't know is how much they can contribute to blood sugar control and weight loss. To the extent that you can eat more foods that have little impact on your blood sugar and less foods that have greater impact on your blood sugar you will lose weight. As you will see, vegetables are the carbohydrate group that has the least impact on your blood sugar.

Take a minute now and go back to the sweet and starchy carbs graphs and compare those to the following veggies carb graphs. Compare how fast sweet and starchy carbs get into your bloodstream, how

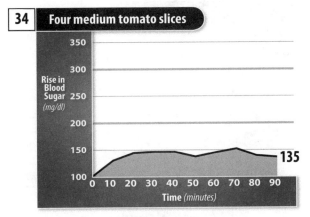

Net blood sugar rise – 35

high they go and finally compare the gray area. The faster a food goes in, the higher it goes, and the greater the gray area the more weight it's going to add.

Cauliflower

Here's an illustration of a very minor impact of fat (butter) when combined with veggie carbs. You can see by the following two graphs that eating cauliflower with butter creates an almost negligible impact on blood sugar and weight gain.

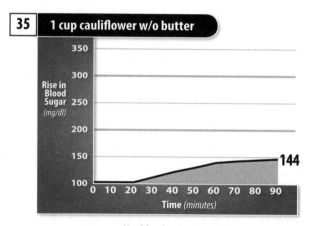

Net blood sugar rise – 44

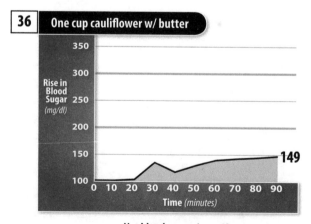

Net blood sugar rise – 49

Asparagus

Asparagus with butter has about the same minimal impact on blood sugar and weight as cauliflower with butter.

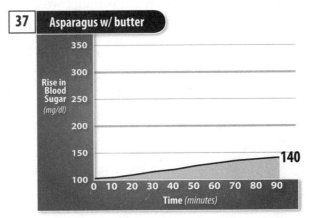

Net blood sugar rise – 40

Broccoli

Once again a vegetable shows its healthy impact. By putting butter on green vegetables you will probably eat more vegetables.

A logical question at this point is what about the impact this extra butter has on cholesterol levels. I'll respond to that question later in this chapter and in the next chapter.

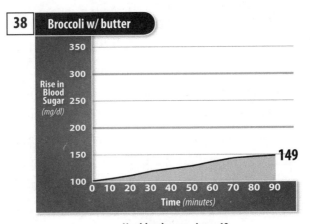

Net blood sugar rise – 49

Carrots

I mentioned "green vegetables" in the last paragraph. Here's a "non-green vegetable, carrots that still performs pretty well. You'll see by the graph that the impact on blood sugar and weight is slightly higher than the previous vegetables but still pretty darn good in terms of small impact on blood sugar and weight.

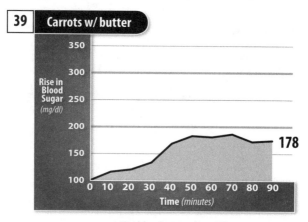

Net blood sugar rise – 78

Corn

When I said "with just a few exceptions, eat more vegetables and you'll lose weight", corn is one of the exceptions. Although corn is considered a vegetable carbohydrate it acts more like a starchy carbohydrate. Take a look at this graph and compare it to the other veggie carbs. Like starchy carbs, corn creates a lot of blood glucose and therefore insulin demand which means more weight gain. Minimize corn in your eating lifestyle.

Potatoes also act more like a starchy carb than a veggie carb. They are a good source of vitamin C and potassium but are also a big contributor to increased blood sugar and therefore weight. If you're trying to lower your blood sugar and lose weight, be cautious of the amount of potatoes you eat. Because corn and potatoes act like starchy carbs, unlike other veggie carbs, putting butter on these two foods will add significantly to blood sugar increases and weight gain.

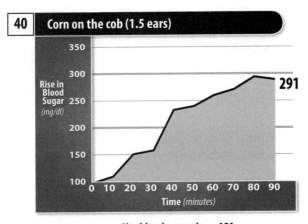

Net blood sugar rise – 191

Conclusions on Vegetable Carbohydrate Group

A very important message from these graphs is that vegetables in general have very little impact on blood sugar and weight gain and that adding butter to vegetables show that has only a tiny impact on blood sugar. Vegetables trigger very little insulin demand so the mixture of vegetables and butter in stomach allow only a very limited amount of butter calories to get into the cells for storage. Over thousands and thousands of tests, I've learned that butter added to vegetable carbs has an insignificant impact on blood sugar and weight. You'll read more about this important point in later chapters.

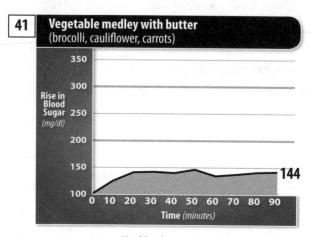

Net blood sugar rise – 44

This is different from adding butter to starchy carbs which trigger—as you've now seen—trigger a lot of insulin demand. All the insulin created by the starchy carbs allows the butter calories to flow into storage cells since the two items are mixed together in the stomach.

I've had so many people tell me that reducing the quantity of food they eat is very difficult and they always feel hungry. One way to solve that problem and lose weight is to eat more of the foods that won't raise your blood sugar much and less of the foods that will. That means eat more vegetables and be free with the butter.

Protein and Fat

I've combined protein and fat because very few common foods are exclusively fat. The two most common foods that derive all their calories from fat are butter (100 calories per serving—all from fat) and olive oil (125 calories per serving—all from fat). Wow, with those calories from fat, they must be bad for you. Right? ... I think you'll be surprised!

Once again compare the upcoming graphs to the sweet carbs, starchy carbs, and fruit juices.

First some breakfast foods comprising protein and fat.

Three Large Fried Eggs
Large eggs have 70 calories each so three eggs have 210 calories, exactly the same number of calories as a Hershey Bar (also 210 calories). Now compare the graphs—a Hershey Bar (graph 4) to the next two graphs, three large eggs (graphs 42 and 43). It very strongly illustrates the point that calories are not always a good indicator of the impact on blood sugar or weight creation. Take special note of the area of gray under the graphs which you know by now is a general representation of weight

gain. It's a good illustration of the value of foods that enter your blood streams more slowly. Remember, the slower the food enters your bloodstream, the more likely you'll burn it before you store it. You'll also note very little difference between poached eggs and fried eggs. For the fried eggs, I used Pam, made with canola, to test them.

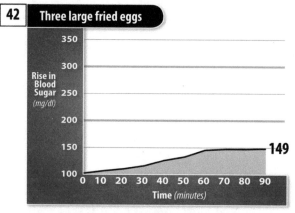

Net blood sugar rise – 49

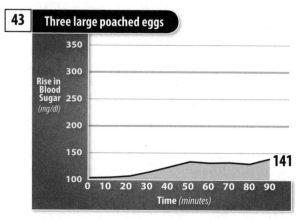

Net blood sugar rise – 41

Bacon

I'm very sure this is going to be one of your biggest surprises. It took me decades to figure out why sometimes bacon seemed to have negligible impact on my blood sugar and sometimes it seemed to have a lot of impact. I finally figured out what created the discrepancy.

After 1000s of blood sugar tests, I stumbled upon the answer to the discrepancy. About 10 years ago I started periodically eating breakfasts with just bacon and eggs or sausage and eggs—no potatoes or toast. I was stunned at how little impact that combination had on my blood sugar. I gave myself less insulin for those breakfasts and started losing weight without even trying to. Since then I have learned that I can add almost any vegetable—with butter—to that combination and similar blood-sugar-lowering, weight-loss will result.

For years whenever I ate bacon and eggs for breakfast, I'd also eat toast and infrequently hash brown potatoes. That mixture of starchy carbs, protein and fat created a very large impact on my blood sugar and triggered the need for a lot of insulin. That large amount of insulin I had to inject allowed all the glucose from that mixture of protein, fat, and starchy carbs to get into my cells for energy and—since the glucose that combination created was more than I could typically burn the largest part went to storage in my fat cells.

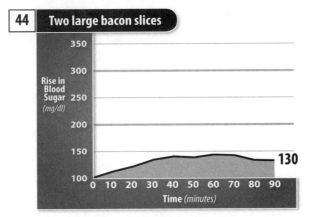

Net blood sugar rise – 30

Compare the bacon graph to the single piece of wheat toast with and without butter (graphs 19 and 20). That comparison provides a good example of the relative contribution to your weight of toast vs. eggs.

Now few people eat bacon alone; I sure don't so following this section on protein and fat, you'll find a section titled, "Good Meals, Bad meals" which will show you which combinations of foods will trigger high blood sugar and weight gain and which will trigger lower blood sugars and weight loss.

So if fat's not the problem, and starchy carbs are, how about heart health and cholesterol? I cover this in much more detail in the next chapter.

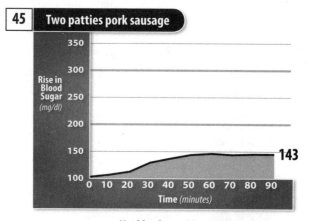

Net blood sugar rise – 43

Rib Eye Steak and Rotisserie Chicken

Here are two more examples of the low blood sugar impact of protein and fat if not combined with starchy carbs.

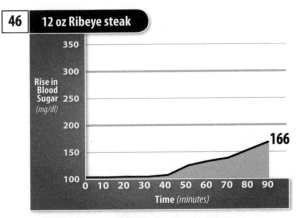

Net blood sugar rise – 66

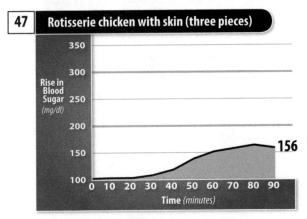

Net blood sugar rise – 56

Halibut and Salmon

Both of these cold-water-fish are excellent choices to keep blood sugar and weight down. In the next group of graphs that "Good Meals, Bad Meals" you'll see how these two fish choices plus Pacific cod can have a significant impact on weight loss.

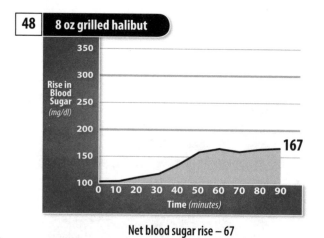

48 | **8 oz grilled halibut**

Net blood sugar rise – 67

49 | **10 oz grilled salmon**

Net blood sugar rise – 43

Cheeses

Most cheese has little impact on blood sugar and weight. They provide a good snack or addition to a meal. I often put a small amount of cheese in a microwave for 30 seconds and melt it for an evening snack.

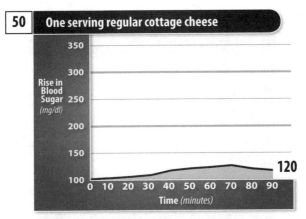

Net blood sugar rise – 20

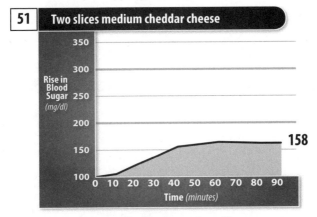

Net blood sugar rise – 58

Cashews and other Nuts

As you can see by this graph of cashews, they don't raise blood sugar by a lot but they are not a free ride. This reflects the impact of 40 cashews which the label says is a "serving". I recommend half that many as a better snack size. Shaved almonds baked on a flat pan and salted make a good tasting and healthy snack.

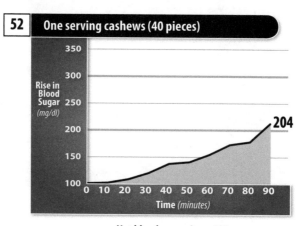

52 One serving cashews (40 pieces)

Rise in Blood Sugar (mg/dl)

204

Time (minutes)

Net blood sugar rise – 104

Good Meals, Bad Meals

Obviously we don't just eat individual foods; we combine them and create meals. You now know that sweet carbs and starchy carbs cause big rises in blood sugar and are big contributors to weight gain. In the following groups of meals, pay close attention to which of the meals have starchy carbs in them and which don't then note their comparative impacts on blood sugar and therefore on weight gain.

Low Blood Sugar, Weight-Loss Breakfasts

I realize that having vegetables with eggs for breakfast is a huge shift in eating lifestyles for most Americans. But if you really care about lowering blood sugar, losing weight, and living a longer, healthier life; breakfast is a great place to start and adding vegetables is a great way to start. Compare these breakfast graphs to the next four breakfast graphs which all have some starchy carbs in them. That should provide some motivation to eliminate starchy carbs and include vegetable carbs in your breakfasts plus you really do have a wide variety of vegetables to choose from just be careful not to include corn and potatoes in your breakfasts.

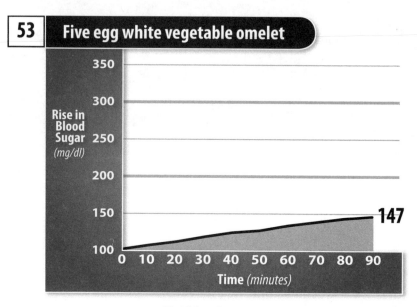

53 Five egg white vegetable omelet

Net blood sugar rise – 47

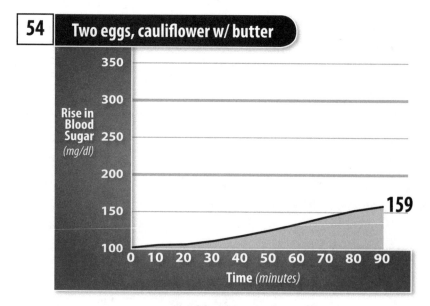

54 Two eggs, cauliflower w/ butter

Net blood sugar rise – 59

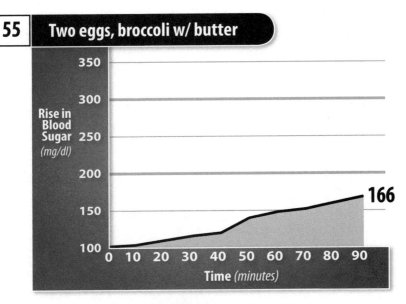

55 Two eggs, broccoli w/ butter

Net blood sugar rise – 66

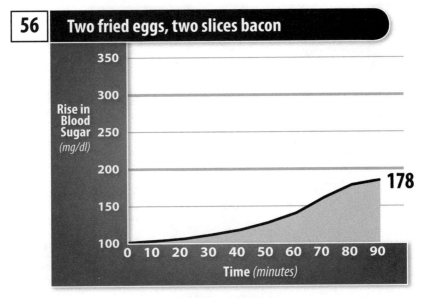

56 Two fried eggs, two slices bacon

Net blood sugar rise – 78

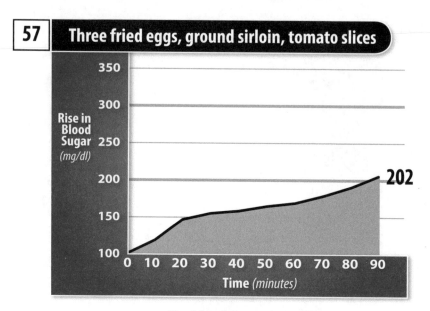

Net blood sugar rise – 102

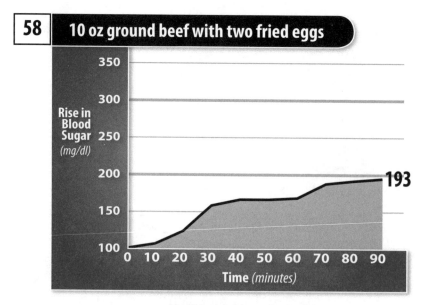

Net blood sugar rise – 93

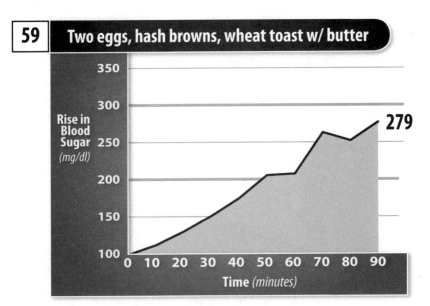

59 | **Two eggs, hash browns, wheat toast w/ butter**

Net blood sugar rise – 179

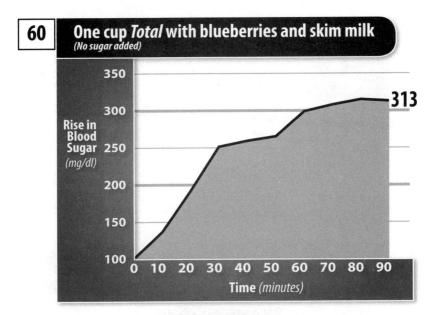

60 | **One cup *Total* with blueberries and skim milk**
(No sugar added)

Net blood sugar rise – 213

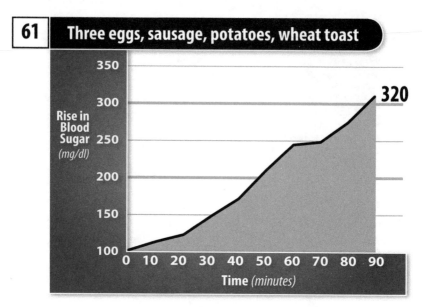

61 Three eggs, sausage, potatoes, wheat toast

Net blood sugar rise – 220

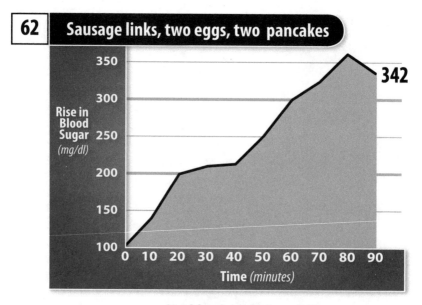

62 Sausage links, two eggs, two pancakes

Net blood sugar rise – 242

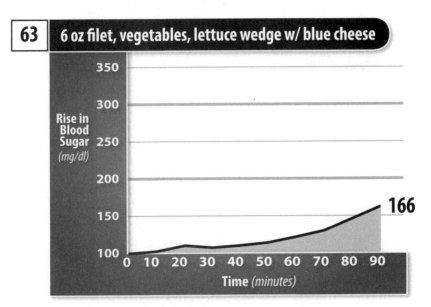

63 | **6 oz filet, vegetables, lettuce wedge w/ blue cheese**

Net blood sugar rise – 66

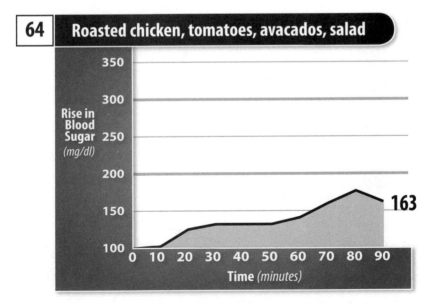

64 | **Roasted chicken, tomatoes, avacados, salad**

Net blood sugar rise – 63

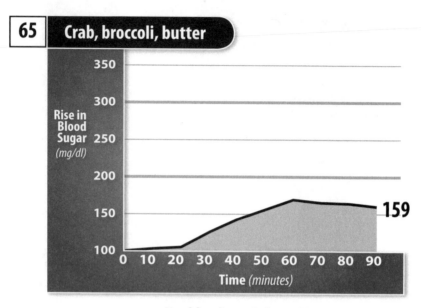

65 **Crab, broccoli, butter**

159

Net blood sugar rise – 59

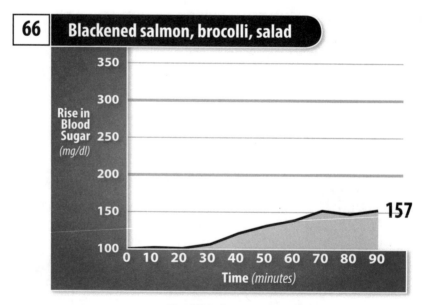

66 **Blackened salmon, brocolli, salad**

157

Net blood sugar rise – 57

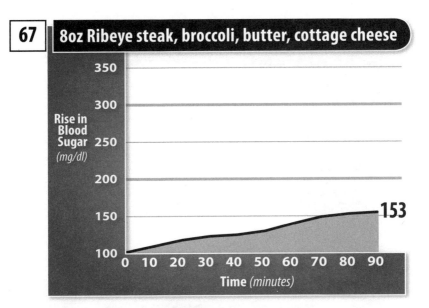

67 **8oz Ribeye steak, broccoli, butter, cottage cheese**

Net blood sugar rise – 53

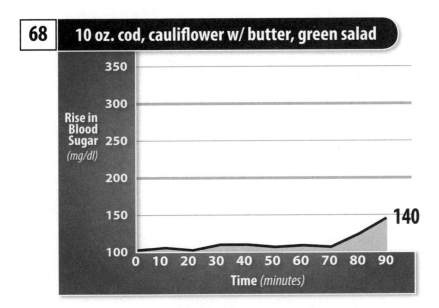

68 **10 oz. cod, cauliflower w/ butter, green salad**

Net blood sugar rise – 40

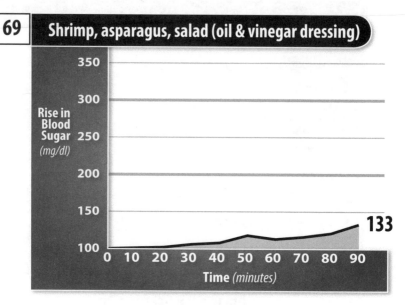

69 **Shrimp, asparagus, salad (oil & vinegar dressing)**

Net blood sugar rise – 33

With the preceding group, notice the absence of starchy carbs. Now compare these graphs with the following *High Blood Sugar, Weight Gain Dinners Graphs.*

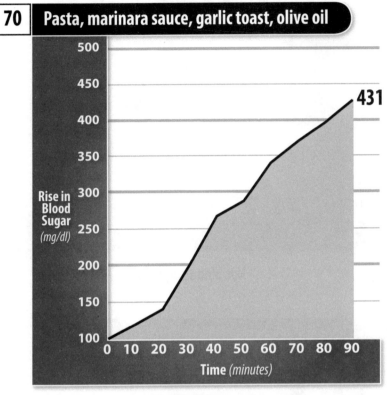

70 **Pasta, marinara sauce, garlic toast, olive oil**

Rise in Blood Sugar *(mg/dl)*

431

Time *(minutes)*

Net blood sugar rise – 331

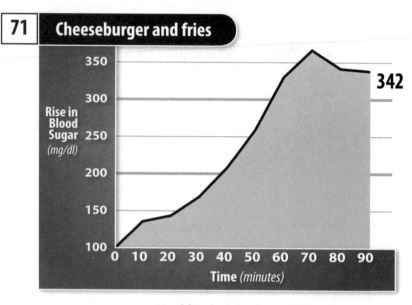

71 **Cheeseburger and fries**

342

Net blood sugar rise – 242

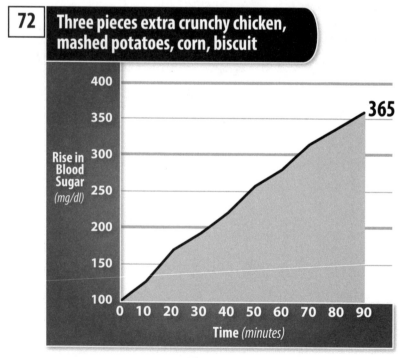

72 **Three pieces extra crunchy chicken, mashed potatoes, corn, biscuit**

365

Net blood sugar rise – 265

Yogurt

I don't eat much yogurt but my testing of original vs. non-fat yogurt further illustrated my conclusions that "It's not fat that makes people fat. It's carbohydrates." Low-fat or no-fat yogurts always list fewer calories and less fat than original or traditional yogurts. So it must mean that low-fat or no-fat yogurts will create less blood sugar increases and less weight gain. Right? Here, take a look.

So why do these graphs show that you'll gain more weight with no-fat yogurt than with original yogurt even though the no-fat and low-fat varieties have less calories. It's because the no-fat and low-fat varieties have more carbs. If they take out the nine-calorie-per-gram fat and replace it with five-calorie-per-gram carbs, the calories will go down. But the issue is not the number of calories it's the type of food. These graphs illustrate beautifully that more carbs and less fat is the problem. Less carbs and more fat is the solution. So give up that bad tasting no-fat yogurt and enjoy the better tasting original or traditional yogurt.

In the next chapter you'll learn the specific steps you can take to create your healthier eating lifestyle.

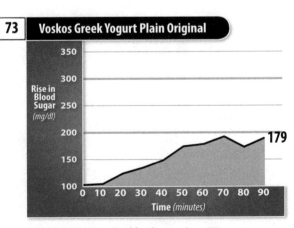

73 Voskos Greek Yogurt Plain Original

Rise in Blood Sugar *(mg/dl)*

179

Time *(minutes)*

Net blood sugar rise – 79

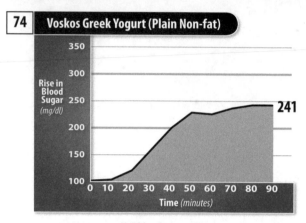

74 | Voskos Greek Yogurt (Plain Non-fat)

241

Net blood sugar rise – 141

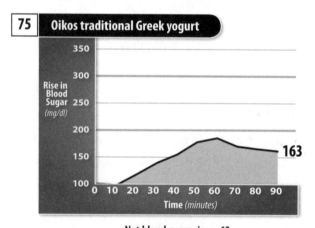

75 | Oikos traditional Greek yogurt

163

Net blood sugar rise – 63

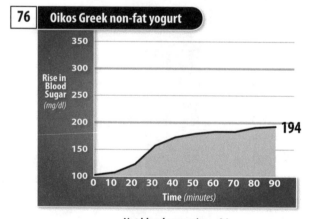

76 | Oikos Greek non-fat yogurt

194

Net blood sugar rise – 94

Blood Glucose and Weight

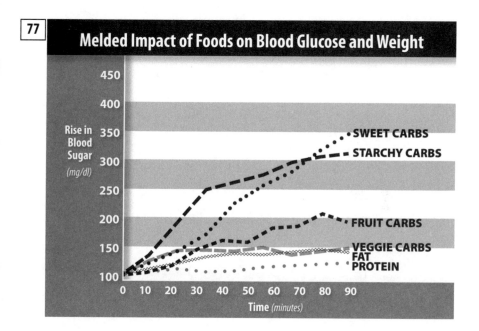

77

Melded Impact of Foods on Blood Glucose and Weight

Rise in Blood Sugar *(mg/dl)*

450
400
350
300
250
200
150
100

• SWEET CARBS
• STARCHY CARBS
• FRUIT CARBS
• VEGGIE CARBS
  FAT
  PROTEIN

0 10 20 30 40 50 60 70 80 90

Time *(minutes)*

This graph illustrates in general terms the food categories of the foods in the graphs that you have just reviewed. It simplifies your eating plan. You can see that the two categories of foods you should *minimize* significantly are SWEET CARBS and STARCHY CARBS. They are big contributors to high blood sugars and big weight gain.

Conversely you'll see that you can *maximize* the VEGGIE CARBS, FAT, and PROTEIN you eat with little impact on blood sugar and weight. Finally you'll see that FRUIT is in the middle and should be eaten in *moderate* portions to avoid a significant impact on blood sugar and weight gain.

AUTHOR'S NOTE:

Review Chapter 5 to help you recall which foods fit into each of these six categories.

Chapter 7

Protein, Vegetables, Fat, and Fruit — The Good Guys

Now that you've had a chance to study the graphs, let's review the key points that you need to lock in your mind.

Sweet Carbohydrates

We now know this category of foods enters your bloodstream very quickly and causes very large increases in blood sugar and therefore weight. Many of these sweet carbohydrates will show up on my blood sugar tests in two or three minutes. The simple sugars with no fat mixed in are the quickest to enter the bloodstream: sugared soft drinks, Skittles, jelly beans, and other candies that are pure sugar. Baked desserts such as cakes and pies usually have some fat in them, as do chocolate candy bars and ice cream. As you now know, fat enters your bloodstream more slowly, so when fat mixes with sweet carbohydrates in your stomach, the combination is a little slower to enter your bloodstream than sweet carbohydrates by themselves, but the result is usually a huge rise in blood sugar and a major contribution to weight. But sweet carbs and sweet and starchy carbs combined enter your bloodstream so fast and result in so much blood glucose that most of it is stored before it is used. That, as we now know, is bad.

Starchy Carbohydrates

You can see from the graphs that this is also a category of carbohydrates that raises your blood sugar very quickly and results in an increase as great as that of sweet carbs. Although most people realize that sweets are big contributors to weight gain, very few realize how much starchy carbs contribute to our national obesity and Type 2 diabetes problem. Starchy carbs may be even bigger contributors to our overweight problem because people in general eat a larger volume of starchy carbs than of sweets. The best step you can take to lower your blood sugar and reduce your weight is to dramatically minimize your consumption of starchy and sweet carbohydrates.

In Dr. William Davis' excellent book, *Wheat Belly*, (Rodale, 2011), Dr. Davis came to conclusions very similar to the conclusions I've come to. He first introduces the problem with what I call starchy carbs with the following headline on the back cover of his book, "DID YOU KNOW THAT EATING TWO SLICES OF WHOLE WHEAT BREAD CAN INCREASE BLOOD SUGAR MORE THAN TWO TABLESPOONS OF PURE SUGAR CAN?"

Early in his book he describes what he calls wheat belly. "A wheat belly represents the accumulation of fat that results from years of consuming goods that trigger insulin, the hormone of fat storage. While some people store fat in their buttocks and thighs, most people collect ungainly fat around the middle."

Once again this is consistent with my message that the foods that trigger the most insulin are the foods that raise your blood sugar the most and contribute the most to weight gain.

Dr. Davis also talks about the lethargy and drowsiness that results from eating wheat based foods for breakfast (I use the term starchy carbs) instead of protein and fat. He states, "I couldn't help but notice that on the days when I'd eat toast, waffles, or bagels for breakfast, I'd stumble through several hours of sleepiness and lethargy. But eat a three-egg omelet with cheese and feel fine".

In his book he also refers to the success that he has had with his patients who replaced wheat based foods with other healthier whole foods, "After three months, my patients returned to have more blood work done. As I had anticipated, with only rare exceptions, blood sugar (glucose) had indeed often dropped from diabetic range (126 mg/dl or greater) to normal. Yes, diabetics became nondiabetics. That's right: Diabetes in many cases can be cured—not simply managed—by removal of carbohydrates, especially wheat from the diet. Many of my patients lost twenty, thirty, even forty pounds."

Two items in that quote deserve a response. First, when he talks about diabetics becoming non diabetics, I'm sure he is referring to Type 2 diabetics. Second, I don't advocate the removal of all carbohydrates from a diet. I advocate dramatically limiting sweet carbohydrates and starchy carbohydrates; vegetable carbohydrates don't need to be limited at all and fruit carbohydrates just need to be slightly limited.

Fruit Carbs

Fruit carbs vary quite a bit, but the graphs should have helped you understand their general impact. The basic message regarding fruit carbohydrates is that they will raise blood sugar a little more than veggie carbs and protein but way less than sweet or starchy carbs. Fruits include many vitamins and water-soluble fibers that are very important to general good health. Including fruits as part of your eating lifestyle is important; however, in my experience fruits such as pineapples, oranges, watermelons, peaches, bananas, and strawberries will raise blood sugar fairly fast and need to be eaten in moderation in order to maintain lower blood sugars and lose weight.

Fruit juices are a different story. They are problematic in causing very fast and very big blood sugar increases and significant weight gain. In many cases a large glass of apple juice, orange juice, or pine-apple juice for breakfast will put on more weight than all the rest of your breakfast combined and it gets into your bloodstream much faster than you can use it. So it gets stored in and on your body.

An Associated Press article from the December 11, 2011 edition of the Honolulu Star Advertiser substantiates what I learned decades ago. The headline stated, "Apple juice is far from nutritious, experts say"… . "nutrition experts say apple juice's real danger is to waistlines and children's teeth. Apple juice has few natural nutrients, lots of calories, and in some cases, more sugar than soda. It trains a child to like very sweet things, displaces better beverages and foods, and adds to the obesity problem. "

In my personal experience, apple juice, orange juice, and pineapple juice all make my blood sugar skyrocket and require me to take much more insulin than the fruits themselves require me to take. In the next chapter, I talk about the steps I have taken regarding juices and rec-ommend those steps to you.

Veggie Carbohydrates

As you could see in the graphs, vegetable carbs are an excellent group of foods for lowering blood sugar and losing weight. Not only do these foods have lots of nutrients but they also enter your bloodstream more slowly than the previous three categories. This means that you can burn the calories from these carbohydrates before they get stored as glycogen in your liver or as fat around your body. For insulin-dependent diabetics it also means that insulin injections or infusions can keep up with these foods' entry into the bloodstream and blood sugar control will be better.

These are the foods your mom told you to eat. She was right. They include most vegetables with the exception of the starchy ones I mentioned earlier. My favorite veggie carbohydrates are asparagus, broccoli, tomatoes, cauliflower, artichokes, spinach, cabbage, carrots, peppers, mushrooms, beets, sauerkraut, and salad greens. I pretty much eat all vegetables but draw the line at lima beans. "No thank you."

Proteins

Protein has gone in and out of favor many times in the past 60 years. From my experience over the past 30 years of blood sugar testing, protein is a very positive part of my diet and weight maintenance. Protein has very little effect on my blood sugar and a very noticeably positive effect on my muscle growth when I match protein with strength training, which I'll discuss in chapter 11.

As you could tell from the graphs, protein will cause neither a quick nor a significant rise in blood sugar. Consequently, I freely eat large quantities of protein with a barely measurable effect on my blood sugar.

Examples of protein that I eat often and freely are salmon, halibut, cod, trout, shrimp, and scallops. I also often include chicken, turkey, and Cornish game hen in my protein-eating patterns and will eat beef, ham, and pork as a change of pace.

My core protein food is salmon (wild, not farmed). I eat it two or three times a week in the summer and maybe once a week in the winter. It's an almost perfect food. With minimal impact on my blood sugar, it's absorbed slowly so the small amount of glucose it creates is burned as fast as it goes into the bloodstream and doesn't get stored as fat. Salmon is also very high in protein and high in omega-3 fatty acids (which all my reading indicates is a good fat). Salmon is also a good source of vitamin D. All that and it tastes great too, as long as you don't overcook it.

In Defense of Fats

I spend a lot more time talking about fats in this chapter than about any other of the remaining food groups because my personal experiences and conclusions are significantly different from what our government through the Department of Agriculture has told us for so many years. Because of that it will take a lot of convincing and repetition to help persuade my readers of the insignificant contribution of dietary fat to your body fat. So please bear with the repetition in my discussions of fat.

The impact of fats has been the biggest surprise to me over my years of testing—maybe revelation is a better word—and I think the same will hold for you. You can see from the graphs in the previous chapter that adding butter to vegetables has almost no blood sugar impact, that bacon alone has minimal impact, that eggs alone with the yolk have almost no blood sugar impact. I probably add more butter to my foods than 99 percent of Americans, and have for 30 years, but I eat very few baked desserts so I don't get all the butter that is used as an ingredient in those foods. Because most of my butter is used on vegetable carbs, my blood profile and cholesterol ratios are great. Remember the words of Dr. John Mues, a friend of mine and a very fit and athletic 60-year-old, "Fat is your friend."

To summarize, I agree with John except I'd call fat a "conditional friend." Fat is your friend if you eat it with protein, with vegetables, or with salads. But if you eat a meal with a piece of fatty meat and have potatoes with butter, or biscuits with butter, then the starchy carbs will create such an insulin demand that much of the fat will flow into the fat storage cells along with the starchy carbs.

The second condition to avoid if you've had fat in your meal is to follow up with dessert. It's similar to the starchy carb effect. The dessert will create such an increase in insulin that the fat you've eaten prior to dessert will flow along with the sweet carbs into the storage cells. So fat is your friend as long as you don't mix it with starchy or sweet carbs.

Here are some examples of foods that have a significant amount of natural "fats": butter, eggs (with the yolk), pork, sausage, bacon, prime rib, most steaks (especially rib eye), hamburger, bratwurst, mutton, and veal (which I don't eat because of the bad treatment of calves).

As I said in the lead-in to this section, fats are not the villains they are made out to be. For years we've read over and over about losing weight with low-fat diets. We've read about low-fat this and low-fat that. Who argued? It seemed so reasonable. If you don't want to be fat then don't eat fat. Simple right? No…wrong.

Think about this for a minute. If eating fat makes people fat, one would think that it might hold true for animals too. After all, enough similarities exist between mice and humans that mice are continually being tested by scientists to see how humans might react to the same food, medications, or environmental situations.

Let's take cows, for example. Do cows eat fat? No. They're herbivores, grazers and foragers of grass and alfalfa. I'd call grass and alfalfa "veggie carbohydrates for cows." Cows, like all other herbivores, naturally develop fat without eating any fat. Up until the early 20th century, cows primarily grazed on grass and alfalfa, but over the last 100 years in America, the beef industry has learned how to make cows grow as fat as possible as fast as possible. How do they do it? They raise cattle in feedlots on a diet of manufactured grain consisting primarily of corn. Remember, corn is one of the few vegetables that act like starchy carbs. I'd call corn "starchy carbohydrates for cows." So in our context, the cows were switched from veggie carbs to starchy carbs and what a difference that has made in the speed and amount of fat accumulation on cows. How often have you heard or read the term "pure corn-fed beef." Corn-dominated grains give beef a juicier, fattier, and tastier texture and they do this very fast. This is great for the beef industry and for all of us who like a tasty, juicy steak once in a while, but is this what you want—to get as fat as possible as fast as possible? Cows get this way almost exclusively on corn-dominated grain (starchy carbohydrates). So would you if you let starchy carbs dominate your eating.

If you are one of those rare Americans who are underweight and want to gain weight fast, this is how to do it. Eat lots of starchy carbohydrates. Throw in lots of processed foods often loaded with starchy carbs and finish off each meal with sweet carbohydrates. But don't waste your time trying to gain weight by eating a lot of natural fats because it's not going to happen.

What Some Others Say About This Approach

The best-known advocate for a general low-carbohydrate diet is Robert Atkins, who in 2002 wrote Dr. Atkins New Diet Revolution. Some of his reasoning was different from mine, and he didn't break down carbohydrates into the categories that I believe are so important to weight loss and good diabetes control.

I recently saw a clip from an interview Dr. Atkins had many years ago with Barbara Walters. In this interview she said to him, "Are you telling me that I can eat as much fat as I want and won't gain weight?" He simply and emphatically said, "Yes, as long as you don't eat that fat with carbohydrates."

My conclusions are just slightly different but significant in impact. Fat will add to your weight if you eat it at the same meal that you eat starchy or sweet carbs. But if you eat only protein and veggie carbs in a meal, you can put all the butter you want on the vegetables—except for corn and potatoes—and it will contribute almost nothing to blood sugar or weight gain. That is, in fact, a very significant difference because it shows that you can eat vegetable carbohydrates with butter or other fat and it will have very little impact on your blood sugar or weight. But if you eat butter, for example, with bread, rice, spaghetti, corn, or potatoes, or if you follow a meal with a dessert (sweet carbs) then that butter will contribute significantly to weight gain. That aside, I do agree with many of his conclusions.

Dr. Eric Westman, director of the Duke Lifestyle Medicine Clinic and one of the authors of A New Atkins for a New You, has been studying low-carbohydrate diets for 12 years and says, "…when it comes to protein and fat, eat as much as you want. You don't have to use portion control. Your hunger will go down when you start eating this way—all you have to do is stop eating when you're full." He also says "Say good-bye to pasta, rice, bread, and corn" among other weight contributors.

My testing generally confirms what Dr. Westman is saying. Once again, the only place where we disagree is that you can put butter, dressing, cream cheese, or sour cream on vegetable carbohydrates and still have the same weight-loss effect.

In an article by Lisa Davis in the February 11, 2011 issue of Reader's Digest, she writes about Gary Taubes' new book, Why We Get Fat—And What to Do About It._Taubes is an award-winning science journalist.

Davis writes, "If obesity researchers are so smart, why are we so large? After all, public health authorities have been hammering home a very simple message for the past 40 years. If you don't want to be fat, cut the fat from your diet. And in those years, obesity rates have gone from 13 percent to 22 percent to, in the last national survey, 33 percent.

"Taubes thinks he know why: Obesity experts have gotten things just about completely backward. If you look carefully at the research, he says, fat isn't the enemy; easily digested carbohydrates are. The very foods that we've been sold as diet staples—fat-free yogurt, plain baked potatoes—hold the butter—and plain pasta—hold the olive oil, sauce, and cheese—actually reset our physiology to make us pack on the pounds. And the foods that we've been told to shun—steak, burgers, cheese, even the sour cream so carefully scraped from that potato—can help us finally lose the weight and keep our hearts healthy."

Taubes continues with his message under the heading "High Fat is Better for Your Heart." Regarding the low-carb, high-fat diet he says, "Your HDL [the good cholesterol] goes up, which is the most meaningful number in terms of heart health... . Not only does your cholesterol profile get better, your insulin goes down, your insulin resistance goes away, and your blood pressure goes down."

He continues, "The low-fat diet that people have been eating in hopes of protecting their heart is actually bad for their heart, because it's high in carbohydrates. The public health effort to get everyone to eat that way is one of the fundamental reasons that we now have obesity and diabetes epidemics."

In 2007, Taubes published *Good Calories, Bad Calories: Challenging the Conventional Wisdom on Diet, Weight Control and Disease*, a book that led the New York Times to assert that "Gary Taubes is a brave and bold science journalist" who shows that "much of what is believed about nutrition and health is based on the flimsiest evidence."

Taubes' message: Political pressure and sloppy science over the last 50 years have skewed research to make it seem that dietary fat and cholesterol are the main causes of obesity and heart disease, but there are, in fact, few or no objective data to support that hypothesis. A more careful look (Taubes researched his book for five years; its 450 pages include 60 pages of footnotes) reveals that the real obesity-epidemic drivers are increased consumption of refined carbohydrates, mainly sugar and white flour.

Bottom line: "Carbohydrate is driving insulin is driving fat deposition." So when it comes to accumulating fat, carbohydrates are indeed "bad calories," as they are the only ones that boost insulin and make fat accumulation possible.

So what's the scientific weight-loss solution? Taubes asserted that since the fewer carbohydrates we eat, the leaner we will be, our diets should emphasize meat, fish, fowl, cheese, butter, eggs, and non-starchy vegetables.

Conversely, we should reduce, or preferably eliminate, bread and other baked goods, potatoes, yams, rice, pasta, cereal grains, corn, sugar (both sucrose and high-fructose corn syrup), ice cream, candy, soft drinks, fruit juices, bananas and other tropical fruits, and beer. Excluding carbohydrates from the diet, he said, derails the insulin peak/dip roller coaster, so one is never voraciously hungry, making weight loss and healthy-weight maintenance easy. "When you eat this way, the fat just melts off."

"Sugar Tied to Fatal Heart Woes"

On February 5, 2014, the *Anchorage Daily News* ran an Associated Press Article by Lindsey Tanner. The headline was **"Sugar tied to fatal heart woes."**

The article said the American Centers for Disease Control and Prevention studied over 30,000 American adults with an average age of 44. Lead author Quanhe Yang called the results sobering and said it's the first nationally representative study to examine the issue.

The article stated, "'Scientists aren't certain exactly how sugar may contribute to deadly heart problems, but it has been shown to increase blood pressure and levels of unhealthy cholesterol and triglycerides; and also may increase signs of inflammation linked with heart disease,' said Rachel Johnson, head of the American Heart Association's nutrition committee and a University of Vermont nutrition professor."

I think within a few years, this type of research will also identify starchy carbs as contributors to those same heart problems, elevated cholesterol and triglycerides caused by sugars. This is just one more bit of support for my argument that it's elevated glucose that is the major contributor to these problems. It's not fat—unless of course the fat is accompanied in your meals by sweet or starchy carbs.

Excerpt from Brad Lemley, DrWeil.com News

> *One of the best books I've found on blood sugar control and health is Dr. Bernstein's DIABETES SOLUTION by Richard K. Bernstein, MD. It's very clearly and persuasively written by a doctor who has lived with Type 1 diabetes for "65 years and counting." Here's what he says about the insulin-fat connection that I've been talking about in this chapter. "The primary source*

of body fat for most Americans is not dietary fat but carbohydrate, which is converted to blood sugar and then, with the aid of insulin, to fat by fat cells. Remember, insulin is our main fat-building hormone. Eat a plate of pasta. Your blood sugar will rise and your insulin level (if you have Type 2 diabetes or are not diabetic) will also rise in order to cover, or prevent, the jump in blood sugar. All the blood sugar that is not burned as energy or stored as glycogen is turned into fat. So you could, in theory, acquire more body fat from eating a high-carbohydrate fat-free dessert than you would from eating a tender steak nicely marbled with fat. Even the fat in the steak is more likely to be stored if it is accompanied by bread, potatoes, corn, and so on."

Dr. Bernstein uses the words "in theory" when he talks about acquiring more body fat from a fat-free dessert than from a "steak nicely marbled with fat." My graphs just showed you that it's not just "in theory." It's reality.

"Mr. President, Take Down That Pyramid"

Certainly our more sedentary, digitally dominated lifestyle has an impact on our collective weight gain, and as a nation we need to be more conscious of our slide into sedentary softness. Although our diminished physical activity contributes to our national weight problem, it's not the biggest contributor. The biggest contributor by far to our national weight gain is our American eating lifestyle.

Thousands of books have been written about what foods to eat in order to lose weight and be healthier. They can be brain-filling, mind-numbing, and flat-out wrong. Most of these books can be traced back to information that has been provided by the United States Department of Agriculture's Food Pyramid. While most of us may only refer to the USDA Food Pyramid maybe once every 10 years, if that, the information it provides does creep into many books and articles that influence our eating habits. If you google USDA Food Pyramid, you'll get 366,000 versions and explanations of it in a quarter of a second. It's America's eating bible and it's wrong.

The USDA says we should eat more than twice as much—six to 11 servings daily of the "bread, cereal, rice, and pasta group"—as any other group including vegetables and fruit. They also recommend eating three times more of the "bread, cereal, rice and pasta" group than the protein group: "meat, poultry, eggs, fish, and nuts." Not only is this wrong. It's almost completely backwards. If I followed their guidelines, I wouldn't be able to sit close enough to my desk to type this book. I'd have to rest the keyboard on my stomach.

No wonder two thirds of Americans are overweight or obese. They've been influenced, whether they know it or not, by the Federal Government's grossly wrong dietary guidelines. What on earth is the government thinking—six to 11 servings daily of the bread, cereal, rice, and pasta group? That's exactly the food group that causes Type 1 diabetics' blood sugars to skyrocket, Type 2 diabetics' pancreases to wear down, and nondiabetics to become overweight or obese. When the government first started publishing its healthy-eating pyramid, less than 20 percent of Americans were overweight. Now, 40 years after they told us how to eat, the number of overweight Americans is approaching 70 percent of our population.

Some say the USDA is influenced by wheat, grain, and corn farming and processing lobbies. That sounds plausible but I don't know. What I do know is that the information it publishes in its Food Pyramid is wrong and contributes greatly to America's overweight and obesity problem. So, "Mr. President, please take down that pyramid."

Now that you understand what you need to eat to better control Type 1 diabetes, to cure Type 2 diabetes, and to lose weight, the next chapter will tell you how by introducing to you, the *Diabetes Lifeline Diet*™.

Chapter 8

The *Diabetes Lifeline Diet*™

Creating a Healthy Eating Lifestyle

In the last three chapters, you learned a lot about what foods will help promote weight loss and what foods will not. Many "healthy diet" books not only miss the target on understanding which foods are best for losing weight, but also don't go beyond just the listing of foods and suggestions for recipes. But that's not the whole story. *Losing weight and becoming healthier is about changing lifestyles. It's about setting new patterns of eating, activities, and sustainable exercise and then making those patterns into habits or lifestyles. Of those three lifestyles, the most important is how you eat.*

Once you start the eating patterns of the *Diabetes Lifeline Diet*™, you will start losing weight right away and continue losing weight until you've reached your ideal weight. At first you'll have to think about it every day. It won't be hard now that you know which foods to eat and which to avoid, but it will take some discipline. Once you follow these patterns for a couple of months, the patterns will become habits; then you won't even have to think about them.

When you wake up in the morning, you don't look at a note that says, "Brush your teeth, wash your face." You don't need to think about

getting a cup of coffee, getting the newspaper from your p
having your normal breakfast. You just do it. And you certair
need a note that says, "Say good morning" to your husband
You've established certain patterns or lifestyles and they've just
become habits.

This is what you'll learn in chapters 8-11: the eating patterns that
will help you start losing weight and the lifestyle habits that will keep
it off for the rest of your life. By way of warning, once you've reached
your desired weight, don't go back to your old eating lifestyle; just
increase the portion size of the better food that you are now eating in
your *Diabetes Lifeline Diet™*.

How the *Diabetes Lifeline Diet™* is Organized in this Chapter

The way I've chosen to organize the *Diabetes Lifeline* changes to get
you on the lifetime path to a healthier life is to first separate *eating in*
from *eating out*. Then I've subcategorized the actions by *breakfast,
lunch, dinner,* and *after dinner*. Two actions don't fit neatly into those
categories: snacking and alcoholic drinks, so I've added an *other* section at the end.

Here's how the balance of this chapter is organized:

Eating In	Eating Out	Other
Breakfast	Breakfast	Snacking
Lunch	Lunch	Alcohol
Dinner	Dinner	
After Dinner	After Dinner	

Breakfast

Fruit is okay but dilute your fruit juice

You saw in chapter 6 how fast and how much orange juice and apple juice raised my blood sugar and consequently would have increased my weight over the years if I hadn't taken the action I'll recommend to you. This action is *diluting your juice*. Some people, as I do, only have juice in the morning but many of you may drink juice at different times throughout the day thinking that it's the healthy thing to do. It's not. The impact on your blood sugar and weight counteracts the positive benefit you may get. Though I didn't include pineapple juice in the graphs, it's very similar to orange and apple juice in its impact.

The way to get some benefit from the vitamins that are present in juices is to dilute your juices before you drink them. In the morning I fill about ¼ of a juice glass with the juice we buy and fill the rest with water. My "go-to" juice is V-8 juice diluted with Pelligrino's Sparkling Mineral Water. I'll use a full-size glass and put about one to two inches of juice in and fill the rest with water. You will be surprised how easy it is to get used to the more diluted juices. It won't take long before full-strength orange juice feels very thick and very sugary.

The benefit you reap from this change will depend on how much juice you currently drink. If you're a big juice drinker, the benefit will be great. A good example of a huge benefit comes via Barbara Mee, a longtime friend and former special assistant to the late Senator Ted Stevens. Barbara had heard me speak about diabetes quite a few years ago. Among the tips I suggested in that speech for losing weight and controlling blood sugar was to dilute juices.

Barbara's husband, Vince, worked in street maintenance for the Municipality of Anchorage. His work at that time involved driving snowplows in the winter and driving trucks the rest of the year. Vince was a bit overweight at the time and thinking he was being very conscientious about his health, he would start his day with a big 20-ounce mug of orange juice in his plow. Many days he refilled the mug at midday and finished it off by quitting time.

Soon after Barbara told him about my orange juice suggestion, Vince coincidentally had a doctor's appointment. He told the doctor about my advice and the doctor strongly agreed. According to Vince, the doctor told him he needed to lose weight and the first thing he should do was "get off that orange juice. That's like mainlining sugar." Vince immediately quit drinking it on the job and cut way back to just a little diluted orange juice for breakfast. Barbara said within months Vince had lost "20 to 25 pounds solely by cutting back on the huge amount of orange juice he drank."

Now both Barbara and Vince are enjoying a well-deserved and active retirement in Florida. They're playing golf together five or six days a week and Vince has never regained the weight he lost after cutting way back on orange juice.

Eliminate or Dramatically Reduce Toast, Muffins, Potatoes, and Bagels for Breakfast

For so many years, many health-conscious people thought eating some toast with jelly, a bagel with cream cheese or a muffin was a decent, healthy breakfast. Not so. In terms of weight gain let's look at those three choices.

Toast and English muffins

If you can't eliminate them, at least eat small portions, like one piece of toast and half of a muffin. But if you eat two pieces of toast that's double the starchy carbs. And if you add jelly or jam that's another 30 calories of sweet carbs that will get into your bloodstream so fast that unless you run to work, you won't burn it before it will get stored in the liver as glycogen and then later on your stomach, legs, or hips as fat.

Cinnamon and Sugar vs Jam or Jelly

If you must have a piece of toast in the morning, do yourself a favor and put a mixture of sugar and cinnamon on it instead of jam or jelly. What— sugar? Yes, cinnamon and sugar. Years ago I had a feeling that jelly on my toast had a bigger impact on my blood sugar than cinnamon and sugar. I started experimenting with my blood testing and found out it was true. So I quit using jelly or jam and started using cinnamon and sugar on my toast and found that my insulin demand went down.

As an experiment, I put the same amount of cinnamon and sugar that I put on my toast into a teaspoon. It turned about to be ½ teaspoon. Figuring the sugar was about 50% of the mixture, I was putting about ¼ teaspoon of sugar on my toast. At 17 calories per teaspoon of sugar I was adding a little more than 4 calories to my toast; compare that to 32 to 36 calories that jelly added. Some would say it's not a big deal; it only saves about 30 calories a day. I'd say look at it this way. That simple, small daily action would save 210 calories a week, which is the number of calories in one Hershey bar. Putting jelly or jam on your toast every morning instead of cinnamon and sugar is equivalent to eating 52 Hershey bars in a year. This is such a good illustration of how making a little change in a daily habit can add up to a meaningful weight loss in a year. Of course it's much better if you just don't eat toast at all.

Bagels and Cream Cheese

Bagels are big. Bagels are starchy and they will be converted to glucose and enter your bloodstream faster than you will typically burn the calories. So eliminate them from your breakfast. If you can't completely eliminate them, eat no more than a quarter of one for breakfast. More cream cheese and less bagel is better for you for two reasons: (1) The more starchy carbs you eat the more the fatty content of the cream cheese will be stored rather than eliminated, and (2) the fat content of the cream cheese will mix with the fast-acting starchy carbs of the bagel and will slow down the bagel's absorption. That slowing of the absorption means your body will produce less insulin and you'll burn more of the calories before they're stored as fat. Even though the cream cheese adds some calories, the real issue is whether you can burn those calories before they are stored. The cream cheese will help you do that. By the way, the same goes for butter. On the rare occasion that I eat toast for breakfast, if I put butter on my toast (which I do) it slows down the speed of absorption of the toast, which balances my insulin input better than without butter. But if you're really serious about lowering blood sugar and losing weight, get the starchy carbs, including cereal, out of your breakfast.

Eliminate Cereal from Your Breakfast Pattern
Remember when we were kids? We'd wake up and pour ourselves as much cereal as would fit in the bowl, put lots of sugar on it, maybe a banana, and then go out and play for three or four hours. If you're going out after breakfast and going to play for three or four hours, go ahead and load up on cereal. But if you're not, you've got to cut back on cereal *and* oatmeal. Just look at the charts one more time.

Again it's the starchy carbohydrate issue. Unless you're going to be very active after breakfast, the cereal will be stored faster than you will burn it and it will trigger storage of the fatty content of your blood. You're much better off cutting out cereal and adding some eggs, some vegetable, and some breakfast meat—if you wish—to your breakfast pattern. Once again the protein and fat in the egg and meat option will slow down the rate of absorption and allow you to burn the small amount of glucose before it ever gets stored.

Do Not Eat Sweet Carbohydrates for Breakfast

I'm sure most of you don't do that but if you do, you really need to stop for the sake of your blood sugar control, your weight, and your health. Review the charts in chapter 6 and see how much a single medium cherry Danish raised my blood sugar in 90 minutes.

Eat More Protein for Breakfast

If you're cutting back on all of the above, then what *should* you eat for breakfast? The answer is eat more *protein* and don't worry about the fat that comes along with it. The breakfast that I recommend starts with eggs. My preference for breakfast is either two or three eggs boiled or poached—without toast—I will almost always add a vegetable—most often cauliflower—to my breakfast and put butter on the vegetable.

Now when should you eat an egg-white omelet and when should you eat a whole-egg omelet? I'll eat an egg-white omelet if I'm going to do a strength workout because an egg-white omelet usually has the whites of six or seven eggs—that means 42 to 49 grams of protein, whereas a full-egg omelet usually consist of three complete eggs, and has only 21 grams of protein. Second, on the rare occasion that I have toast or potatoes with my eggs, I'll always have an egg-white omelet and never accompany it with bacon. Remember, the fat in the egg yolk or with bacon will have almost zero impact on your blood sugar or weight as long as you don't eat any starchy carbs with them.

When I say that fat will not significantly add to your blood sugar or weight as long as you don't eat starchy or sweet carbs with the meal, here's more specific timing. *Based on my blood sugar testing, I've learned that I should not eat starchy or sweet carbs one hour before a meal with fat in it, during a meal with fat in it, or three hours after the meal with fat in it.*

Eat Vegetables for Breakfast

Who eats vegetables for breakfast? The truth is not many Americans do unless they are making a veggie omelet or a fritata. But we're

missing out on a great health addition for our first meal. 1
eating toast and started eating tomato slices for breakfast y
Then I moved into different vegetables. Now I almost alway ....c a
healthy portion of asparagus, broccoli, cauliflower, or carrots all with
melted butter. Once I started that habit I started losing weight quickly
even though that wasn't necessarily my goal. Like the fat in bacon and
eggs, the butter fat will have little impact on your blood sugar. Switch-
ing away from starchy carbs for breakfast and to protein and vegetables
with or without butter is one of the easiest and most effective ways
to reduce blood sugar and lose weight. I choose to use butter with my
vegetables because they taste so much better and my daily consumption of vegetables goes way up.

In Summary, do this for Breakfast

⟶ Dilute your juices.

⟶ Eliminate starchy carbohydrates such
    as bread, muffins, cereal, and potatoes.

⟶ Do not eat sweet rolls, donuts, or any
    other sweet carbohydrates for
    breakfast.

⟶ Eat more protein and fat.

⟶ Start adding a vegetable to your breakfast.

If you start that eating pattern you will start losing weight very
quickly because the glucose from those foods will go very slowly into
your bloodstream and you'll burn that glucose before it's stored around
your body in all the places you don't want it stored: mostly stomach
for men and legs and hips for women. The other benefit of a breakfast
with more fat, protein, and veggie carbohydrates is that it's still

entering your bloodstream by lunchtime. That results in a much more diminished sense of hunger at lunch than you would have if you had just eaten cereal, bagels, or any other starchy carbs. So you will be less likely to eat a big lunch.

Lunch at Home

Minimize Starchy Carbs for Lunch

Once again do everything you can to minimize bread, buns, rolls, macaroni, and pasta, and cut out desserts with lunch.

Eat Plenty of Protein, Fat, and Veggie Carbs for Lunch

Don't worry about holding back on protein, fat, or veggie carbs for lunch. Remember a salad consists mostly of veggie carbs and you can put dressing on the salad with near impunity as long as you don't eat any starchy carbs (including croutons) or have any sweets just before lunch, during lunch, or for three hours after lunch.

Most people already know how good most vegetables are for you but I'll repeat again what most people don't know that's even better. Veggie carbs are so slow to enter your bloodstream as glucose that you are very likely to burn that glucose before it's ever stored. Protein is also absorbed slowly and fat is the slowest of all foods. It's one of the reasons that most diabetic regimens don't even recommend counting grams of protein or fat—and they shouldn't count grams of vegetable carbohydrates. These three groups for lunch will help you eliminate snacking in the afternoon and leave you less hungry by dinnertime. Enjoy as much as you want from those three groups.

By following this *Diabetes Lifeline* pattern I described for breakfast, you won't be as hungry at lunchtime and by following the pattern I described for lunch, you won't be as hungry at dinnertime. That also means you'll be less likely to snack after these meals.

I do realize that it isn't always a sense of hunger that dictates whether we snack or not. Often we snack just for something to do. I talk about this later in the chapter on activity.

Fruit is Okay for Lunch

If you follow my suggestions above but do have fruit with your lunch, it will be a slightly bigger blood sugar and weight contributor than the protein, fat and vegetables that you have. So don't have too much. But if fruit is your biggest weight contributor for lunch you're going to do just fine and continue to lose weight.

Eliminate Dessert after Lunch

Most desserts are combinations of sweet and starchy carbs such as cakes and pies or sweet and fatty carbs such as ice cream. Remember those combinations are blood-sugar-raising, weight-gaining bombshells.

Dinner at Home

Now you'll see that I don't recommend eating fatty foods as freely for dinner as I do for breakfast or lunch because fat takes as long as three hours to get into your bloodstream. That's good for breakfast and lunch, because the fat goes in so slowly that you can burn it in your daily activity. But if you eat dinner too late, the glucose from the fatty foods will be going into your body while you're sleeping and that, of course, is not good. You burn so little glucose while you sleep that most of this glucose won't be used. It *will* be stored.

Dinner is the meal that is the biggest contributor to blood sugar elevation and weight gain for a number of reasons. In America, dinner has traditionally been the biggest meal; it's the meal that is least likely to have its calories burned by post-meal activity, and it's the meal most likely to have dessert associated with it.

I was eating dinner with a friend last week and he said, "Look at you. You don't even have to think about what you eat for dinner." My answer was short and quick. "I've been thinking about what I eat for dinner for 30 years." It's true. I rarely sit down for dinner and just "dig in." At meals I'm always thinking about minimizing starchy carbs, sweet carbs (dessert), and at dinner I also think about minimizing fat. The key word here is *minimizing*, not eliminating.

We all desire some starchy carbs at times and we're all going to have desserts once in a while. But the important issue—that you're now aware of— is the huge impact that they will have on your blood sugar and on your weight. Think of it this way. If the price of gasoline were to go up by two dollars a gallon tomorrow, we probably wouldn't just flat out stop driving but we would be much more cautious about how much we would drive and every time we got in our car, the impact on our pocketbook would likely be on our minds. So think about starchy carbs and sweet carbs like that. We're all going to eat them once in a while but when you do always think about the impact on your blood glucose and weight. Just keep minimizing the portions every day until it becomes part of your *Diabetes Lifeline* habit.

If we're having a special dinner with warm, aromatic rolls being passed around the dinner table, I'm going to have one—with butter, of course, even though I know that's bad for me. If we're having company for dinner and a desert is served, I often will have a small to portion. These small enjoyments are an important part of life. I haven't given them up and you don't have to either. But remember— make them special, not part of your regular dinner routine.

So what should you eat for dinner? The good thing about breaking down foods into the six groups instead of just three is that I can tell you which food groups you can maximize with minimal impact on blood sugar and weight and which food groups you should minimize. Once you're able to recognize which foods are in which groups, losing weight and keeping it off will be much easier.

Based on thousands of after-dinner blood sugar tests here a...
foods and actions for lower blood sugar and weight loss at dinn...

Eat Dinner As Early As You Reasonably Can

The earlier you eat the better the opportunity to use the glucose in your bloodstream for energy rather than for storage. In the activity chapter I'll talk about how much my insulin demand is reduced by some small activity such as walking around the yard, going out to the store or other similar activities will burn. More activity after dinner is, of course, better but even a small amount will make a difference as you will learn later.

Eat Plenty of Protein and Veggie Carbs

Fish, poultry, and veggie carbohydrates should be the core of your dinner. You can certainly add red meat to your dinner if you choose. Just be sure to eliminate starchy carbs.

At home I have typical dinners of grilled, blackened, baked, or very lightly breaded Alaskan salmon, cod, halibut, or fresh trout from the lake we live on. Crab and shrimp are also two of our favorites. Both have almost negligible impact on blood sugar and weight. Our veggie carbs are typically broccoli, cauliflower, asparagus, green beans, and a variety of mixed salads with lettuce, vegetables, nuts, and fruit. Maybe three or four times a month we'll have chicken instead of fish and a few times a month we'll have steak.

I make a special point of saying "typical" dinners and not "every" dinner because we all want special dinners on occasion. That's simply an important part of life. Don't give those times up. Enjoy them but even on those special times don't go overboard on starchy carbohydrates or desserts.

Fruit Is Fine for Dinner or after Dinner

As you now know, fruit raises blood sugar more than protein, vegetables, and fat; but for most fruit that difference is not significant.

Fruit does have a lot less impact on blood sugar than sweet carbs and starchy carbs; that difference *is* significant. So go ahead and have fruit with or after dinner if you choose but don't overindulge and don't put the fruit on ice cream—sorry to tell you that.

Reduce Portion Sizes for Dinner

Portion size for dinner is more important than portion size for breakfast and lunch. It's the meal you're least likely to burn and most likely to store as fat simply because you usually will not have as much activity after dinner as you have after breakfast or lunch. At first you'll find it hard to think about dinner as a small meal. As a child and a teenager at home I remember my dad would finish a big dinner, typically of fried chicken, roast beef, or meatloaf with mashed potatoes and gravy, often with corn and biscuits and then lean back in his chair and declare with great satisfaction, "I feel like a million bucks." It was his way of saying he was full and being full was good.

You may have grown up with the same messages I heard every day. "Take all you want but eat all you take." "Clean your plate." "Eat your potatoes." The intent was all positive but when you heard it over and over you couldn't help but think eating a lot is good and not eating very much is bad.

I still remember vividly the first time I asked for a second helping of potatoes—a food I never liked as a kid. I was 12 years old and as soon as I asked for the second helping, Dad fell out of his chair and ended up on the floor (on purpose, of course). He made such an impression on me with his dramatic demonstration that I still remember it 58 years later. His message was, "Eating potatoes is good, the more the better." As you now know, potatoes aren't necessarily healthy, and for dinner I want to add the message that more isn't always better and full isn't always good.

If you can adopt a mindset that really full after dinner is not necessarily good and feeling somewhat satisfied is better, you'll be well on

your way to improving your blood sugar control, losing v
sleeping much better. I know this is not easy but if you can s
smaller dinners your pattern, it will eventually become your habit.
You'll slip and backslide a little as you start making dinner a smaller
meal. Don't say, "I failed and can't do this." Promise yourself you'll do
better tomorrow.

Here are two suggestions for starting the habit of "dinner as a
small meal."

1. Make a promise to yourself to eat your dinner for one month
   from a dessert plate. This will constantly remind you of your
   goal to make dinner a smaller meal. If you can do that for one
   month, you'll find yourself eating less and feeling better right
   away. When you feel you know what a smaller dinner is and
   when you think you can continue eating smaller even if your
   plate is bigger, go back to a normal dinner plate. You'll find a
   feeling of pride as your dinner plate actually has spaces
   among your helpings of food.

2. Start making a checkmark for each day you're successful in
   making dinner a small meal. Maybe the first week you'll be
   successful for only three dinners out of seven. The next week
   shoot for four or five days of success with your new pattern.
   Keep on doing that until you've succeeded all seven days in a
   week. Then shoot for a second consecutive week of that
   pattern. Once you get to four consecutive weeks, *you'll be very
   close to making small dinners your habit.*

Eating the types of food I recommend in smaller portion sizes will
not only help you start losing weight and gaining control of your blood
sugar right away, but more importantly, it can become a healthy eating
habit that will help keep you lean and trim for the rest of your life.

There is a danger, however, in smaller dinner portions. The temptation to snack after dinner and before you go to bed will be even greater. How can you deal with that temptation?

After-Dinner Snacks

I've talked about breakfast, lunch and dinner and of those three meals, dinner is the meal most likely to contribute to weight gain and blood sugar problems. But right up there with dinner as a big contributor to weight gain is what's eaten after dinner—evening snacks.

Like dinner, an evening snack is a habit that is less likely to be followed by activity. So when you're snacking after dinner you're contributing mightily to blood sugar increases and weight gain. After years and years of testing my blood sugar after dinner while sometimes snacking and sometimes not, here are six conclusions I've arrived at.

1. After-dinner snacks are bigger contributors to weight gain and blood sugar increases than are postbreakfast and postlunch snacks. This may be an obvious conclusion simply because we're all more likely to burn some glucose from snacks we eat at 10 a.m. or 3 p.m. than snacks we eat at 8 or 9 p.m. Those late-evening snacks are more likely to be stored than burned. I've never been in the habit of eating a midmorning or midafternoon snack and I don't recommend either but they are not as impactful on weight and blood sugar as a postdinner snack.

2. If you are going to snack after dinner, stay away from ice cream or potato chips. They will not only raise your blood sugar (and weight) because of the sweet and starchy carbs, but also, because of their fat content they will both continue to increase your blood sugar for three or more hours after

you eat them. By that time, you're likely going to be asleep and subject to the worst-case scenario of increasing blood sugar while you're burning very few calories and therefore subjecting yourself to the worst possible blood sugar and weight gain combination.

3. If you feel you must snack, the best by far is a veggie selection or some protein. My favorite veggie snacks are broccoli, cauliflower, carrots and radishes with blue cheese dressing. The dressing is okay as long as long as you don't have any starchy carbs such as crackers with it. For protein snacks, I like smoked salmon, shrimp, or reindeer sausage.

4. A good way to improve your snacks is, "Don't buy the bad stuff." If you do buy ice cream, potato chips, candy, and similar snacks and you keep them visible and handy in your freezer or pantry, *you will eat them*. It's easier to resist them at the grocery store than to resist them in your home.

5. My next suggestion is to ask yourself when you're most likely to eat sweets. I'm guessing it's when you're watching TV or in front of your computer. Before you sit down, ask yourself what else you could snack on besides sweets. Right now as I'm writing this, I'm snacking on walnuts my wife roasted for a salad yesterday. Even with the healthier snacks I suggested in the last paragraph, do not eat them by the handful. Eat them one at a time and take a little time in between. I've learned over the years to eat snacks less frequently and more slowly and savor each bite a little more. By doing that you will automatically be eating a little less. It's a good pattern to get into and soon you'll find it has become a habit.

6. The best plan of all is *not to snack after dinner*. If you can accomplish that you will have taken one of the biggest weight loss and blood-sugar-lowering steps possible.

In chapter 10 I talk about being more active between dinner and bedtime and how that not only burns glucose and lowers insulin demand but also helps decrease the likelihood of snacking after dinner.

Applying the *Diabetes Lifeline* to Eating

Breakfast Out

Stay Away from the Softball-Size Muffins

I'm talking the ones you see in coffee shops, bakeries, and supermarkets. Stay away from them. A bite now and then won't hurt, but most of those muffins could easily serve a whole car pool or a book club. Not much good to say about those muffins except if you do want to put on weight, that's a good place to start. You'll also be hungry in two or three hours and will be likely to snack again before lunch. The same goes for sweet rolls or donuts.

Stay Away from Breakfast Cereal

As you now know, these foods will cause higher blood sugars and much more weight gain than eggs will. Combined with toast, they are very bad for anyone trying to lower blood sugar or lose weight.

Order Whole Eggs with Yolks Under these Conditions

If you haven't ordered any starchy or sweet carbs for your breakfast, you're okay eating whole eggs. But if you've ordered any toast or potatoes you should go with an egg-white omelet or egg-white scramble.

Presuming no starchy carbs, your best whole-egg options are vegetable omelets, vegetable frittatas, or just plain eggs with a vegetable. And if you don't have starchy carbs you can have bacon with little impact on blood sugar or weight.

Order Egg Whites under These Conditions

If you're in a workout pattern and want to increase your ratio of muscle to fat, you should eat egg-white omelets or frittatas. Remember that typical egg-white omelets in restaurants have the whites of six eggs, which means 42 grams of protein, whereas a whole-egg omelet usually consists of three whole eggs and gets you 21 grams of protein.

The other times you should order egg-white omelets are when you choose to have toast or potatoes; that's when you need to avoid the fat in the yolks of eggs. The toast or potatoes are going to provide the openings for the yolk fat to join all the glucose they have created as it flows out of the bloodstream into the fat storage cells.

My staple for breakfast in restaurants for the past 15 years has been egg-white omelets. I usually do have one piece of wheat toast with butter but very rarely do I order potatoes. I often ask for tomatoes or avocados instead of potatoes.

The slice of wheat toast keeps it from being a perfect breakfast like I have at home with eggs and vegetables, but it's a pretty good breakfast. Nobody is going to eat perfectly. I sure don't and you don't have to either. But if you follow the advice in this book, you'll do great.

Breakfast at Fast-Food Restaurants

For a fast-food breakfast, I recommend an Egg McMuffin at McDonalds—not the whole meal, which includes potatoes fried in corn oil, just the sandwich. To cut down on starchy carbs, I just eat half the bun. If I'm on my way to play golf or go fishing, I'll order two but still just eat half the buns. As a bonus McDonald's also has really good coffee.

A number of fast-food restaurants including Subway are offering healthier breakfasts. Whenever you can, try to figure out a way to eat less of the starchy carbs that usually come with the breakfasts.

Lunch Out

Good Lunch Choices at
National-Franchise Sit-Down Restaurants

As you begin lowering blood sugars and losing weight by cutting back on starchy carbs and adding protein, vegetables, or salads, here are some thoughts on restaurant options.

Here's my suggestion for a healthier lunch technique if I'm eating in franchise restaurants like Chili's, TGIF, Appleby's, Red Robin and so forth. I'll order a hamburger, a fish sandwich (not breaded), a chicken sandwich, or a turkey sandwich, or pastrami. I'll always ask if they have an alternative to French fries. If they don't, then I'll do without the fries. Once French fries make it to your plate, they will also make it to your mouth. Most of the time, however, you will be able to get a vegetable alternative. It's an opportunity to have another helping of some vegetable. When you get your food, take the top off the sandwich and set it aside. Use your knife and fork to eat the meat, chicken, turkey, pastrami, or fish and the onions, tomatoes, and lettuce in the sandwich, then leave the bottom half of the sandwich on your plate. By leaving both halves of the bun behind, you've contributed greatly to lowering blood glucose and losing weight.

This, of course, also holds true for lunch at any other restaurant that serves lunch. I just used national-franchise restaurants because of their standardized menus.

Fast-Food Restaurants

Like most people I find myself at fast food restaurants once in a while. For me that's three or four times a month. For some it may be as much as seven or more times a week. Eating too often at fast food restaurants can be a problem but not necessarily. Here are my recommendations for ways to eat fast foods that will keep your blood sugar, insulin demand, and weight down.

Arby's

Arby's has a large roast beef sandwich that I really like. Here's my pattern for eating it. I always ask for one of their plastic forks. Then I sit down, take the top half of the bun off and just eat the roast beef and when I'm done I throw both halves of the bun away. That has very little impact on my blood sugar or insulin demand. I'm always amazed at how they can make roast beef so juicy.

Carl's Jr

Carl's Jr. has a low-carb hamburger that's one of my favorite fast-food burgers. It's simply their standard burger wrapped in lettuce instead of a bun. That diminishes dramatically the impact it has on my blood sugar, insulin demand, and weight. It's a little big so I don't always eat it all and be careful about trying to eat it in your car. It can be a little messy. I usually sit down in the restaurant and eat it there. You get a lot of meat and you won't be hungry again until dinner.

Subway

Subway offers a lot of choices. Now that you know about veggie carbs and protein you can use that information in your selections. My pattern is to always order the six-inch instead of the 12-inch. Then, as I do with most fast-food sandwiches, I just eat one half or none of the bun.

A General Review for Eating at Fast-Food Restaurants

If you just remember a few points when you're eating at fast-food restaurants you'll do your health a big favor:

Cut back on the buns, the bread, the tortillas, and the taco shells. It can be a little inconvenient but eating only half or less of these blood-sugar-raising, weight-adding, starchy carbs should be a part of your fast-food eating pattern.

Cut way back on all foods breaded with cornmeal or deep-fried in a corn oil Jacuzzi. Yep. That means French fries, onion rings, fish, or chicken. You should cut them out completely but if you don't, then figure out your own method to cut way back. Share an order with a friend or better yet, two friends. Ask for a half order or (gasp) throw half of your order in the trash can. Better to put it in a trash can than in a stomach that doesn't need it.

If you can completely cut out starchy carbs then you can add all the protein, vegetables and fat to your lunch that you want. But if you can't cut out starchy carbs completely then more protein and vegetables and less bun is a compromise formula. The protein, whether in the form of fish, chicken, or hamburger will also be a contributor to muscular growth or maintenance.

Mexican Restaurants

Most Mexican foods as prepared in Mexican restaurants in America have a lot of fat, starchy carbs and some protein as primary ingredients. If you do eat in a Mexican restaurant it's better to eat there for lunch than for dinner. You'll have more time to burn off the large amount of glucose that will result. If you can order something like fajitas, that has the protein and vegetables separated and easily eaten without having to eat the starchy-carb wrappings, you should do that. That's very tough though, because it takes away from the enjoyment of that food. Also cut way back on the refried beans and rice as they are very starchy and will have a big impact on your blood sugar and weight.

In general, Mexican-American food is good, it's inexpensive, and it's fast, but be aware of the big contribution to blood glucose and weight.

Dinner Out

Portion Size—the Biggest Problem in Most American Restaurants

About 10 years ago I had flown down from Alaska to visit my mom in Southern California. Instead of flying home after the visit, I decided to do something a little different and take a train, the Sunset Limited, from Los Angeles to Seattle and then fly home to Alaska from Seattle. As the train rolled north through the hills of the San Joaquin Valley, I sat down at a nicely set table in the dining car for lunch and was joined by a Dutch couple. They had been touring America by auto and were now taking the train to Seattle to catch a flight home to Holland.

They were very pleasant, congenial, and open people, but unfortunately I've forgotten their names so I'll just call them Mr. and Mrs. Holland. I asked them the obvious question, "What's your impression of America?" With no hesitation, Mrs. Holland blurted out, "Big." I said, "Big? Well, yes America is a big country." She said, "No, it's not just the country—it's everything. Everything's big." I knew they had talked between themselves about this because Mr. Holland continued her thought. "The mountains are big. The roads are big. The cars are big. The people are big, and the food in the restaurants is big."

Well, I'd never heard anyone call restaurant food "big" but they continued laughing and describing a litany of the large portions of food that they had been served at the last half dozen restaurants they had patronized along their journey. In the years since that conversation, I've become more sensitive to portion sizes in restaurants and often discussed it with Mary. The Dutch couple was absolutely correct. The portions in restaurants are very, very big.

If you eat in restaurants a lot, cutting back on the portion sizes, eating fewer starchy carbs, and ordering dessert only for special occasions, not as part of every meal out, are essential patterns you need to start and turn into habits if you want to lose weight.

By now you know the general guidelines for what to eat. So I'm going to focus on portion size, which I believe is the biggest problem for most of us when we eat dinner out.

Here are three effective ways to reduce portion size in restaurants:

1. Share the entrée with your dinner partner. This idea is becoming fairly common especially with restaurant dinner customers in their 50s and older, but it's a good idea for anyone of any age who wants to control blood sugar and lose weight. Some restaurants will, however, charge a second-plate fee but many do not.

2. Make an appetizer (or two) your dinner following the *Diabetes Lifeline* guidelines you now know. If you try this for a few months as a pattern and are able to let it evolve into a habit, you will have achieved a great health victory and be on your way to better blood sugar control, significant weight loss, and dramatically improved health. Make no mistake about this. It is hard. Your need to ask yourself how badly you want or need the positive results you will experience.

3. As you place your order, ask the server to put half the meal in a to-go container *before he or she brings it out to you.* You'll find it so much easier to only eat half of the overly generous plateful of food if you don't see the other half until you look in the refrigerator the next day.

Mary and I learned another interesting technique for eating smaller dinners from Joan Rivers. Although we haven't adopted her specific technique, we have used her basic premise in another way. During my second term as mayor, we were invited to a small dinner at the Captain Cook Hotel in downtown Anchorage to welcome a group of well-known television personalities who had come to Anchorage for the Iditarod Dog Sled Race.

The dinner was hosted by Mary Lou Whitney and her husband, John Hendrickson, whose family has been longtime friends with our family. I was only vaguely familiar with some of the guests: Mary Ann Mobley and her husband, Gary Collins; Susan Lucci; and Joan Rivers. All of the women were very petite and looked quite trim for their age. Actually, I don't even know how old they were so I guess it's more accurate to just say they all looked trim and attractive.

The whole group was very congenial and friendly. While I was talking mostly with Mary Ann Mobley, my wife, Mary, was sitting next to Joan Rivers and seemed to be engaged in lively conversation. On our way home from the dinner, Mary told me how delightful Joan was and recalled that she had eaten very little. Because she had eaten so little, Mary asked her if she was okay. Joan answered, "Oh yes, I'm fine. I just ordered my usual predinner meal of diet Jell-O from room service before I came to the restaurant." Joan explained to Mary that she always did that before eating dinner at a restaurant.

Now I'm not recommending a full portion of diet Jell-O before dinner, but it certainly worked for Joan to keep her from being too hungry and it may work for you. We will often drink a glass of Pellegrino Sparkling Water before dinner and I sometimes have a large glass of chicken bouillon in the late afternoon—which my kids and their friends tease me about. We both feel we eat a little less when we do that but it's just a periodic action for us and not a regular pattern.

In conclusion, the biggest problem with dinners in American restaurants is portion size, and you have to solve that problem your own way. But the general food choice guidelines of low starchy carbs and less frequent desserts— in combination with smaller portions for dinner only will show significant blood sugar improvement and weight loss results very quickly.

Chapter 9

Getting Started on Your *Diabetes Lifeline Diet*™

Easy Changes and Harder Changes

Eating Lifestyle Changes—Comparing Degrees of Difficulty to Degrees of Benefit

You'll see in this chapter that some of the lifestyle changes are very easy, some are slightly harder, and some are very hard. You'll also find that the degrees of benefit vary. Some will make a slight difference in your weight and health in the short run but will still be significant in the long run. Other changes will have a bigger benefit right away and will be even more significant over the months and years. And some changes will have a dramatic impact very quickly and will be life-changing over the years.

You'll stumble or falter a bit along the way but the changes will be worth it. Remember, each of these changes is part of the whole package of lifestyle changes that together will give you a healthier life. You don't have to embrace and adopt them all but the more of them you do the healthier you'll be. Nor do you have to be perfect in your eating lifestyle; you only have to be good.

I struggled for a long time on how to present these actions by ease or difficulty of the action and significance of the benefit. Should I assign a number, sort of like degree of difficulty in diving or gymnastics? That didn't work because it implied a degree of specificity that was not defensible. The same applied with the degree of benefit. How do you assign a valid numeric value to the different changes I've recommended? Finally I came up with the idea of an **Diabetes Lifeline Grid**. Along the horizontal axis (X axis) is the *degree of difficulty* and along the vertical axis (Y axis) is the *degree of benefit*.

As you look at the *Diabetes Lifeline* Grid, you'll see that the action in the lower left-hand quadrant of the grid is easy and has fairly modest benefit. Those actions that are higher in that quadrant are more beneficial and those that are farther right are slightly more difficult.

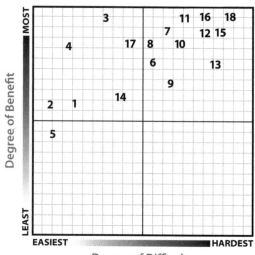

Diabetes Lifeline Grid

Going clockwise from the lower left to the upper left-hand quadrant, you'll find those actions that are still easy and have great benefit in both the short and long term. Focus on these actions immediately. As in all quadrants, the higher they are the greater the benefit and the farther right the more difficult. In the upper right quadrant are the actions that will be harder but will have great short- and long-term benefit. These are the changes that you'll have to work at, but they will be life-changing. Finally, in the lower right-hand quadrant would be changes that are hard and will have little benefit. I haven't even discussed anything that conceivably might fit in that quadrant and would have no reason to do so.

Breakfast

1. Reduce starchy carbs in your breakfast.

2. Eat egg-white omelets if you have any starchy carbs at all.

3. **Eliminate starchy carbs from your breakfast—no cereal, no toast or muffins, no potatoes.**

4. **Add more protein and vegetables to your breakfast—whole eggs and butter are okay if you eat no sweet or starchy carbs.**

5. **Dilute your breakfast juices.**

Lunch

6. Reduce starchy carbs in your lunches and eat more protein and vegetables.

7. **Eliminate starchy carbs at lunch and eat only protein, fat, vegetables, and maybe a small amount of fruit for lunch—butter and salad dressing are okay.**

8. Eliminate desserts at lunch.

Dinner

9. **Eat dinner earlier.**

10. Eat more protein and vegetables and fewer starchy carbs for dinner.

11. **Eat only protein, vegetables, and a small portion of fruit for dinner** (butter and salad dressings are okay if you eat at least three hours before going to sleep).

12. **Reduce portion size for dinner at home and in restaurants.**

13. Share an entree with your dinner partner at restaurants.

14. Order an appetizer—or maybe two— in place of dinner at restaurants.

15. Ask for half of your meal to be put in a to-go box before you get it.

After-Dinner Snacks

16. **Eliminate eating desserts as a regular habit—special occasions are okay.**

17. Improve and/or reduce your after-dinner snacks.

18. **Eliminate your after-dinner snacks.**

AUTHOR'S NOTE:

If you're really serious about losing weight fast, take note of the eating actions I put in **bold type.**

Review the changes listed below and then review the location of each change on the lifestyle graph. After you've considered the benefit and the ease or difficulty of those changes, decide which you want to include in your new eating lifestyle.

If you're really serious about losing weight fast, take note of the eating actions I put in bold type. Your weight loss will start right away and will continue. When you reach your ideal weight, don't go back to your old way of eating—instead, just slide back to some of the nonbolded actions.

A Final Summary of the Food Groups to Lock into Your Memory

Important Note: To review the individual foods that make up these six food groups plus juices refer to the section in **chapter 5** titled **"More Detail on the Six Food Groups Used in this Book"**

Sweet Carbohydrates	Enter your bloodstream very fast, contribute greatly to increased blood sugar and weight, and are generally empty calories with little or no nutritional value. Drastically minimize or completely eliminate these foods to lose weight.
Starchy Carbohydrates	Are also very fast to enter your bloodstream and contribute greatly to high blood sugars and significant weight gain. Minimize or possibly eliminate these foods to lose weight faster.

Fruit Carbohydrates	Enter the bloodstream moderately fast, but for the most part don't cause dramatic increases in blood sugar and weight. Moderate these foods to avoid gaining weight.
Fruit Juices	Cause quick and significant increase in blood sugar and weight. Dilute your juices to lower blood sugar and lose weight.
Veggie Carbohydrates	Enter your bloodstream slowly, have significant nutritional value, and contribute much less to blood sugar and weight gain than starchy carbohydrates, sweet carbohydrates, or even fruit carbohydrates. By eating more of these foods, you'll naturally eat less of the big weight-contributing foods. Eat all you want except for corn and potatoes.
Proteins	Are generally slightly slower than veggie carbohydrates to enter your bloodstream. They provide a significant benefit to muscular development and are so insignificant to weight gain that most diabetic diet regimens don't even advocate counting protein.
Fats	Are the slowest of all food categories to enter your bloodstream. Because of that slowness, fat calories are often used up by your daily activity as they enter your bloodstream and never get a chance to be stored. Just don't combine fat with sweet or starchy carbs.

Revisit the Graphs

To further lock into your memory how fats combined with starchy carbs—as well as sweet carbs—will cause great rises in blood sugar whereas fats combined with vegetables or protein will not, go back and revisit the graphs that show all the food combinations and the complete breakfast and dinner combinations. You'll be reminded of the big impact of fats when combined with starchy carbs but not with vegetable carbs or protein.

If you cut out sweet and starchy carbs, you can eat all you want of protein, fat, and veggie carbohydrates and you will lose weight easily and quickly and without feeling hungry all the time. If you can totally eliminate starchy carbs from at least two meals and minimize them in the third meal, you'll still be amazed at your quick and permanent weight loss and blood sugar normalization.

SECTION III

Moderate Changes to Your Activity and Exercise Lifestyle

For Type 2, Type 1, and Borderline Diabetics or Prediabetics

... and Anyone Who Wants to Lose Weight and be Healthier

Chapter 10

Walking and After-Dinner Activity—Your Best Lifelong Activity Lifestyles

For older diabetics or anyone who wants to lose weight

The Trick with Life Is to Make It Look Easy.

—Anonymous

I've previously explained that three lifestyle changes are important for anyone who wants to lower blood sugar, lose weight, and enjoy better health. I'll repeat them because they are so critical to your success. The three lifestyle changes are : (1) *Adopt a healthy eating lifestyle—the most important of the three lifestyle changes based on my blood sugar tests; (2) embrace a healthy, active lifestyle—the second-most important of the three; and (3) embark on a simple, maintainable, healthy, structured exercise lifestyle.*

The previous section covered the most important of the three lifestyle changes necessary to lower blood sugar, lose weight, and improve your health—*a healthy eating lifestyle.* This chapter covers the second-most important lifestyle change—*an active lifestyle.* Based on blood sugar test and resulting insulin demand, if I do well in the other two healthy lifestyles (eating and a structured exercise program) but am sedentary the rest of the day, my insulin demand is about 10% higher, which translates to a small incremental weight gain. I use the word "small" here because I'm referring to only one day. But all the lifestyle changes I'm proposing are incrementally small but they will be life- and health-changing in a year's period of time and then for the rest of your life.

If you're a Type 2 insulin-dependent diabetic or a Type 2 non-insulin-dependent diabetic who is trying to lose weight without adding activity or exercise to your daily life, you're in for a somewhat more difficult journey than if you can embrace all three lifestyle changes. If you are one who can do it with just a change in eating lifestyle alone—and many can—the best you can hope for is to be lean and a little soft and I don't think that's necessarily what you want.

This chapter is about stepping up the activity level in your daily life in ways you may never have thought of and making those new levels of activity your new active lifestyle. Daily activity is the easiest of the three lifestyle changes to make and the easiest to develop into habits. I'll teach you how to develop this new lifestyle while recognizing that many of you reading this book may have some significant limitations on what you can do now. So we'll start slowly and build from there.

Why So Many Other Nationalities Are Slimmer Than Americans

Over the past 40 years, I've visited urban and rural areas in about 60 countries on six of the world's seven continents (I haven't been to Antarctica), and have come to realize that most of the world's people walk a lot more than Americans do. Some may say that we Americans are lazy. I disagree totally with that premise. It's because of factors far out of the control of most of the world's citizens—primarily the historical development and design of cities and the economic imperatives of countries—that determine whether people walk a lot or don't walk much.

Most European and Asian cities were far along in their development hundreds of years before automobiles replaced horses, oxen, and humans as the primary vehicles for moving goods and promoting commerce. The width of the streets in Europe and Asia was designed to accommodate the needs of the time. Buildings were then built hard on both sides of streets with little room for more than sidewalks and narrow streets for the relatively narrow, slow-moving carts. To adjust for automobiles is now prohibitively expensive and destructive of cities' infrastructure. As a result, the narrow streets remain unaccommodating to automobile driving and parking. The result: people walk.

On Mary's and my first visit to China with Jane Angvik and Vic Fischer in 1980, our interpreters claimed Beijing had only 800 privately owned cars in the whole city of nine million people at that time. The result: millions of people walked or rode in a rolling sea of bicycles on every main artery. Now Beijing has over 20 million people with hundreds of thousands of cars crawling in a perpetual traffic jam, but because of the economic imperative of general poverty, millions of people still walk and ride their bikes.

In Paris, London, Prague, Lausanne, and most other large European cities, the sidewalks are bustling and flowing with walkers. Walking is necessary, of course, but also enjoyable for native citizens and visitors alike. Only Manhattan, in my experience in American cities, comes close to matching the walking requirements and experiences of European cities.

In the African countries I've visited—Malawi, Tanzania, and Zambia—people walk for a different reason. Malawians have few cars and insufficient discretionary income to even dream of purchasing a car or fuel. Walking is the primary form of transportation and commerce. In my mind's eye I clearly see tall, slim, erect Malawian women defining the boundaries of sparsely used dirt roads, walking in single lines with wooden branches, sacks of maize, and jugs of water balanced firmly on top of their heads. This is the commerce of rural Malawi. This is their highway system.

As you can guess, people in the areas I've just described are largely slim and healthy looking. Certainly, other factors may influence their apparent health but I believe walking is a significant contributor. The balance of this chapter will give you techniques to develop a pattern of walking more and making that pattern your lifelong habit.

Buy a Pedometer and Some Good "Around Home" Walking Shoes

One of the best investments you can make for long-term health is to buy a pedometer. Almost any sporting goods or outdoor store will have one and most are less than $20. The pedometer will measure with good accuracy how many steps you take in a day. For the most accurate results, you should attach it to a belt or the waist of your pants or skirt. Also available are more sophisticated digital devices that provide more information than you'll ever need but they still work for our purposes.

I also recommend that you buy what I call "around home" walking shoes. Most of your walking is going to be around home, around the yard, around your neighborhood, shopping and doing errands, so buy shoes that you're comfortable wearing in those venues.

Once you get a pedometer it's important to keep a log of how many steps you're taking. Begin by establishing your baseline—how many steps you're taking now. It's best to do that for at least a week since some days, especially weekends, may vary from weekdays. Then use that baseline to compete with yourself. Each day try to beat the previous day's steps. After you've used it for a couple of weeks or so and have an idea of what you are doing and what you may be able to do in terms of steps per day, then you can start thinking about goals.

Here are some things to think about in your daily-steps goal setting. Dr. Catrine Tudor-Locke published a study in 2004 involving

200 men and women. The men in the survey took an average of 7,192 steps a day and the women in the survey took an average of 5,210 steps.

In 2001, the U.S. surgeon general, Dr. David Satcher issued "The Surgeon General's Call to Action to Prevent and Decrease Overweight and Obesity." The report recommended 30 minutes a day of moderate activity. Most health experts seem to agree that 8,000 to 9,000 steps a day is an excellent, healthy pattern to be in. That may sound daunting, but I'm willing to bet that most of you will be surprised at how many steps you're already taking.

Whether your baseline is 1,000 steps a day, 3,000 steps, 5,000 steps or more, this suggestion is easy and very flexible. At the end of the first month you'll not only feel healthier but you'll also enjoy a feeling of physical pride that you may not have felt for a while.

Find a Friend to Walk With on a Regular Schedule

Finding a friend or friends to walk with is one of the best ways to build a regular walking habit. You'll have both company and commitment. You'll see things in your own neighborhood you never noticed from your car. You may end up stopping and talking to people who have lived near you for years and who you've never shared a story with. People who have enjoyed this habit for a long time talk about this time as a pleasant, satisfying part of their day.

Here are two stories of people in their 60s and 70s who have developed a habit of walking and maintained that habit for over 10 years—and all are healthy and trim.

My Sister, Rosanne,
and Her Walking Friend, Dona Avila

Thirteen years ago, my sister, Rosanne Bader, retired after a 32-year career as a teacher and principal in the Pomona Unified School District. Her friend, Dona Avila, an art teacher in the same district, had

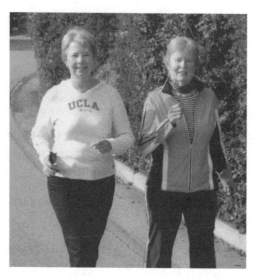

13 Year Walkers

Rosanne Bader on the left, and Dona Avila, have been walking the neighborhood hills in Pomona, California since they both retired from education careers 13 years ago.

retired a few years earlier. Once my sister retired, the two ladies committed to starting a walking program together.

The two women live just two houses away from each other near the top of a hilly area covered with nicely spaced homes fronted with cedar and foothill pines as well as oak, alder, and cotton-woods. For nine months of the year flowering plants decorate their walks.

They made some early decisions about their walks that have served them well. They decided upon morning walks—"We start at 8 a.m.," said Rosanne. "We agreed to a Monday-through-Friday schedule and we simply call each other the night before if a morning meeting or commitment requires a cancellation of the day's walk," she added.

Now, 13 years later, Rosanne talks warmly about their lifestyle habit. "Since our homes are at the top of the hill, we always start out downhill. We like to talk as we walk and at first we could only talk on the downhill half. Coming home uphill we just walked without talking—not because we didn't want to talk, we just couldn't walk uphill and talk at the same time. Now," she says, "we talk the whole way. It's just fun. We greet our neighbors, wave to the cars, and pick up trash along the way. The 2.2 mile up- and downhill walk seems to go by so fast."

It's no surprise that these women are so trim and so healthy. Rosanne, by the way, is 73 and Dona is 78 and both look and feel great.

The Anchorage Trash Fairies

About nine years ago my wife and I moved to a new neighborhood, a few miles from where we had lived for over 30 years. Early in the morning as I was leaving for work or workout, I would often see a group of cheerful, physically-fit neighbors walking, talking, laughing… and picking up litter. I knew some of them and asked how long they had been doing their early morning excursions. Judy Sedwick, apparently one of the leaders, said, "Well I started when my daughter was in kindergarten and now she's 41."

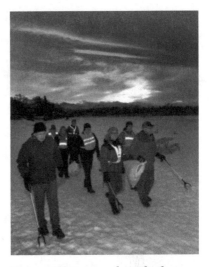

Five mornings a week—whether spring , summer, fall, or winter for about 35 years— this sociable and fit group of Anchorage citizens have been walking our neighborhoods and picking up trash.

They have a good activity lifestyle, they're in excellent physical shape and our little part of the world is better because of them.

The Importance of After-Dinner Activity

At no other time in your day will activity have as much impact on your weight and blood sugar as the hours between dinner and bedtime. This is the time our promises die. This is the time our health gets superseded by sloth unless we actively choose health. This is not just other people's problem. It was mine too for a few years and it may be yours now.

In the early 1990s, I was approaching 50 and I noticed a more sedentary after- dinner pattern showing up in my life during the winter months. The summer months were not a problem because of the excess of daylight. Mary and I were almost always active and busy during those long, sunny summer evenings. In fact, more than once

I recall her saying, "Rick, you'd better stop cutting the lawn, it's almost midnight and you'll disturb the neighbors."

November through April, though, was a different story. I found myself doing what I never thought I would do—surfing the television channels from about 9 p.m. to 11 p.m. It didn't take me long to realize I was not only wasting two hours of my life each night, but I was also increasing my insulin requirement by about 30 percent for the dinner that night. Remember, increasing insulin demand means gaining weight. So I decided to make two changes to my life pattern. The first change was to always have at least 30 minutes of activity between dinner and bedtime. The second lifestyle change was to start going to bed earlier and begin waking up earlier. Both of those changes had a very positive impact on my health, my physique, my insulin requirement, my blood sugar control, and my productivity. Instead of wasting two hours in nonproductive lethargy late at night I went to bed earlier, started waking up two hours earlier and began going to a health club for a light workout first thing in the morning.

Not only did the 30 minutes of activity reduce my insulin demand in the evening and therefore avoid weight gain, but waking up early and working out started a long-term exercise pattern that still continues today.

While I'll talk more about the importance of moderate exercise programs and daily activities in the next chapter, here I'll speak specifically about what you should do after dinner.

When I first began to associate the increasing rise in blood sugar and the resultant increasing insulin demand with lack of activity after dinner, I decided to try experimenting with that premise. I decided the best way to establish the impact or lack of impact of activity after dinner was to eat the same or very similar dinners on consecutive nights and follow those dinners with either activity or inactivity before bedtime. I chose a dinner that Mary and I ate often, and made a special point of trying to eat closely similar portion sizes.

The routine dinner I chose in this experiment was grilled Alaskan salmon, a vegetable with butter, a green salad with nuts and grapes, and one small slice of bread, buttered, with melted cheese on top— I've since stopped eating that.

It turned out my premise was accurate. When I followed that meal with at least a half hour of some activity after dinner such as walking, boating, working in the yard, fishing off our dock, or playing with our grandkids, six to seven units of insulin was sufficient to balance that dinner. If I sat down in front of my computer or our TV set between dinner and bedtime and had virtually no activity, it would take nine to 10 units of insulin to balance that same meal. That's roughly a 30 to 40 percent increase in insulin demand because of my inactivity. You now know that more insulin means more weight gain and less insulin means less weight gain, or weight loss, for the same meal.

Let me explain the impact of that activity in another way. The roughly three units of additional insulin I needed to take when I had no activity after dinner is about the same amount of insulin I would take to balance a standard-size Hershey bar, which is a little more than 200 calories. Not having any activity after dinner was like adding the equivalent of a candy bar to my dinner. Having no activity after dinner every day for a year is like adding 365 candy bars to your calorie intake. If you assume a candy bar is about 200 calories, that's roughly a 75,000 calorie impact over a year. Every pound of fat is equivalent to about 3,500 calories, which means those 75,000 calories added because of inactivity equal over 20 pounds of fat per year.

Now conventional wisdom would say that 30 minutes of light to moderate activity is insufficient to burn 200 calories, but conventional wisdom hasn't been tested like this. My observation is that a continuation effect of calorie burning occurs, and the slight increase in metabolism continues prior to bedtime and for the first hour or more of your sleep.

My conclusion based on the specifics of insulin demand is that some activity between the time you eat and the time you go to bed is the most important and effective activity you will have all day. So how do you get into the habit of doing this?

The first thing you need to do is to get into the mindset of moving after dinner. If you're one of those folks who gets up from the table, moves to the living room and positions yourself in front of a TV or a computer, changing that pattern and adding at least a half hour of some physical movement after dinner will have a big impact on your weight and health.

After-Dinner Activity Suggestions

Do some of your daily "out of home" chores after dinner instead of doing them before dinner. For example, do your food shopping and any other shopping or errands after dinner and when you do it, park farther away from the store than you normally would.

➡ Instead of doing yard work on weekends, do a little bit each evening after dinner.

➡ Get in a habit of taking an after-dinner walk with friends or your spouse. It doesn't have to be long. It can be just around the block to start and let it build naturally to longer walks. This is different from a morning walk. It doesn't have to be as long to be effective in using up the glucose created by your dinner.

➡ If you go out to eat in a location that accommodates walking, get in the habit of parking three or four blocks away from the restaurant and walking to the restaurant. That action means you'll walk before you eat and more importantly, after you eat.

➡ If you have a shopping mall nearby, go there and walk around for a while.

➡ When you do sit down in front of the TV, make it a point to get up and walk around your house or yard during commercials. This will also help you curtail snacking because a commercial break is one of the most common snacking cues.

My point is this. You don't have to have to work hard after dinner, you just have to move. You're going to move naturally after breakfast and lunch but you don't necessarily move after dinner. You should begin this pattern and make it your habit. You will be astounded at the difference this will make in your weight and health over the years.

This Is Not an Activity but It Works— Lower the Temperature in Your Bedroom at Night by a Couple of Degrees

Right! You mean I'm going to lose weight while I'm sleeping? The answer is yes, you will. This is not really an activity but it's an action. Think about it this way. If you heat your house with natural gas and say the temperature is 50 degrees outside, you'll be burning some amount of gas to make up that 20-degree difference to keep your house at 70 degrees. If the next night, the temperature goes down to 40 degrees, are you going to use more gas than the night before to keep your house at 70 degrees because you've got a 30-degree difference to make up? Of course you will.

Your body's like a house—well, actually I hope not—it works hard to keep its temperature at 98.6 degrees Fahrenheit. The greater the difference (lower only) between the ambient temperature outside your body and 98.6 degrees, the more calories your body must burn to heat itself. For example, if you keep your bedroom temperature at 70 degrees, that's a difference of 28.6 degrees your body needs to make up. If you lower your bedroom temperature at night to 68 degrees, your body will have to burn more calories to make up 30.6 degrees.

Now you may put on more blankets to keep comfortable but your face—and in my case my head—will still be exposed. So some extra calories will be burned.

At first I was perplexed by some differences I noted in my morning blood sugars because I'm a believer that all blood sugar levels have a reason behind them. But I couldn't figure out why, when I went to bed with my blood sugar stable (no insulin or food going in) at 110 or 120, I sometimes woke up with a blood sugar very close to that and sometimes with a blood sugar 50 or 60 points lower. It took me years and years to recognize that the drop of 50 or 60 points in my blood sugar was related to the temperature. The lower the temperature, the more glucose I burned and the more my blood sugar dropped.

Of course, 50 points on my blood sugar doesn't exactly relate to 50 calories, but coincidentally, it's close. To give you an idea about what that means in terms of food—for me this is about the amount of weight I'd lose by not eating a third of a typical candy bar or by not drinking a quarter of a can of sugared soda every day. I know that because that's what I would have to eat or drink to raise my blood sugar about 50 points.

Think about this from the converse standpoint. If two people my size (6 feet 3 inches and 190 pounds) lived in adjoining identical apartments and one kept the bedroom at 68 degrees, the other at 70 degrees, the one in the warmer bedroom would pay a weight gain penalty each night of the equivalent of eating a third of a candy bar each day.

You may say, "A third of a candy bar? That's no big deal." But think about the impact it would have over time. A third of a candy bar a day is roughly two candy bars a week or 100 candy bars a year. Now you've got to believe 100 candy bars a year will make a difference in your weight.

This action falls into the category of pretty easy to do, and will have a small short-term impact but a meaningful, cumulative impact over the years. However, if lowering your bedroom temperature negatively impacts your sound sleep, don't do it. A good night's sleep is priceless and this book contains lots of other lifestyle options that will result in weight loss and better health.

Chapter 11

A Moderate, Sustainable Exercise Lifestyle
"The Type 2 Exercise Program"

Primarily for Type 2 diabetics who want to lose weight and possibly lose their dependency on insulin and oral diabetic medications

Also for Type 1 diabetics who want to look and feel healthier and reduce their insulin dosage ... and for any Americans who want to lose weight, feel better and look better

The Importance of a Moderate Exercise Lifestyle

This chapter covers the last of the three lifestyle changes you need to embrace in order to lose weight, get healthier, and become stronger. By way of review, developing a *healthy eating lifestyle* is the most important lifestyle change you can make. Creating an *active lifestyle* and adopting a *structured exercise lifestyle* are the final two lifestyle changes needed to live a long, healthy life.

Your goal should be to start this as a program, make it a pattern, let it evolve into a habit and then make it a continuing part of your lifestyle.

This program, "The Type 2 Workout Program" is designed for Type 2 diabetics who may never have taken part in a structured exercise program or who may not have exercised for a long time. It's a simple, short program that starts out very slowly and nonstrenuously and allows you to match your workout to your strength—or lack of strength—and increase as it fits your ability. As you will see, the key element in this program is never to work so hard that you don't want to do it the next day. I want you to feel good after you complete each daily workout—not worn out.

Although this program is designed primarily for Type 2 diabetics, it will also be very helpful for anyone, overweight or not, who would like to have a simple, structured, sustainable exercise program as part of his or her life.

The beauty of adding this program to your lifestyle is the addition of aerobic health *and* muscular gain.

The aerobic health you'll achieve will be beneficial to your heart, circulatory system, and myriad other benefits you can read about in any one of the hundreds of books about aerobic sports.

The strength-gain element of the exercise program I'm recommending also has multiple benefits. To start with, whether you're a man or a woman, having a higher percentage of muscle than of fat in your body means you'll burn more calories in your daily life than a person of the same sex and size who has less muscle than you do. This means that you can eat the same amount and types of food as this other person and gain less weight or lose more weight than he or she will. Other benefits include increased strength, better posture, and less fragility as you age. And, by the way, you'll look better. You will experience all these benefits by making the strength-training element a part of your exercise lifestyle.

But the real gain for Type 2 diabetics is that this exercise program combined with the first two lifestyles changes I've recommended may completely eliminate your Type 2 symptoms and for all practical purposes make you effectively a nondiabetic. Adding this lifestyle to the other two lifestyle changes could very likely eliminate the need for insulin injections for some Type 2 diabetics and eliminate the need for oral medications for others.

Remember that exercise and activity work like insulin to lower the blood sugar and can diminish or eliminate the need for oral medication or insulin for Type 2 diabetics. Food, of course, raises your blood sugar.

Why this Exercise Program is Different from All the Others

How many times in your life have you heard the terms "Give it your all," "No pain, no gain, "Go the extra mile," or "Don't quit now." If you haven't competed in a lot of sports, you may not have heard these motivational missives at all but believe me they're very common in America and probably many other countries. I see people—mostly guys—every week in gyms living these guidelines. They're pushing heavy weights. They're grunting. They're yelling. They're sweating and—they usually disappear within a few weeks. Not always though. If they're training for a competition, they may be doing the right thing and they may very well persist until the competition. But if they expect it to be a lifetime health and fitness habit, it won't work.

Who This Program is *Not* For

Walk past any supermarket magazine rack and you'll see more than a dozen fitness magazines for men and women. Probably 90 percent of the photos focus on abs (stomach muscles) and all of them have pictures of men and women with beautifully toned and hard, lean muscles with little body fat. Many of the serious muscle magazines show bizarre-looking, overly muscled behemoths. If your goal is to look like these men and women this program is not for you. To look like these magazine cover photos, here's what you would have to do. Pay attention to what I said about food and then add about 200 grams of additional protein to your daily diet. Then find a good trainer and commit to spending about 10 to 20 hours a week in strength and aerobic training. When you've done all that find a photographer who's good at photoshop and can take away the blemishes and any remaining fat.

Who This Program *is* For

However, if your goal is to lose weight, lower your blood sugar, lower your blood pressure, feel better, and look better, this program is for you. Beyond your body looking better, your face will look better as you lose fat. As we gain weight, our faces become rounder and lose the definition we had when we were thinner. As we lose weight, the definition slowly and subtly begins the return trip to our faces.

If you're a woman, in addition to the above, you can expect to reduce your dress size, improve your posture, and cut inches off your hips and legs.

If you're a guy—I've learned I can call a man a guy but calling a women a gal, the parallel equivalent, is mostly trouble—in addition to the above, you can expect to increase the size of your shoulders and chest, decrease the size of your stomach, and improve your posture.

Because this is not an intense program, it will work for any Type 2 diabetic from an overweight preteen to an optimistic 85-year-old grandpa who still wants to chase women even if it's only downhill, or to the 90–year-old woman who, like most of us, still wants to look and feel better.

This is my program. I've used it for the past 15 years and it's worked beautifully. It's simple, clear, easy to start, and easy to maintain. Adding this simple exercise program to the first two elements—a healthy eating lifestyle and an active lifestyle--will result in a complete fitness lifestyle. Starting these lifestyles is the process. Fitness is the result.

The Basics of the Type 2 Diabetics' Workout Program

This Type 2 workout program is designed for people who have not exercised on a regular basis for years or maybe have never exercised.

It's a simple program to get you into a gym and keep you coming back. If you don't belong to a gym or health club or have one nearby, you can still follow the patterns I'm proposing by purchasing some basic— or if you choose, more elaborate—equipment to use at home.

Here's the basic philosophy of the
Type 2 Diabetics' Exercise Program:

1. The program requires and rewards persistence, not intensity. It may be as little as 20 minutes three days a week or as much as 40 minutes six days a week—or somewhere in between.

2. You'll include strength training and aerobics in your daily workout starting at a level appropriate to your existing condition and ability.

3. You'll start slowly and never work so hard on any given day that you don't want to do it again the next day.

4. You'll start every series of repetitions (reps) with weights light enough to allow you to repeat a motion 25 times (25 reps). I'll explain why later in this chapter.

5. You'll never use a weight so heavy that you can't do 15 reps.

6. You should approach this as a one-year program. By the end of that time you'll be a fitter, healthier person and you'll know what works for you, so you can determine your own future program adjustments.

7. As you begin this program, you should increase protein consumption to give your muscles the fuel to grow. Remember, protein has little impact on your blood sugar.

8. If you can maintain this program for three months, you will be well on your way to making it part of your everyday life and a final step in your new healthy lifetime lifestyle.

Getting Started with Your Aerobic Workout

Your aerobic workout is very simple. Most gyms have three or four options and if a gym doesn't work for you, walking or riding a bike can achieve the same goals.

In a gym, your workout can take place on a stationary bike, a treadmill, a stair climber, or an elliptical trainer. Do only what you're comfortable with. You may be able to start by walking for only 10 minutes; that's fine. Remember not to push yourself. This is the beginning of a long, pleasant journey and if you work too hard at first you'll likely make it only a short journey.

If you're using a machine that measures calories you burn, start with a 10- to 15-minute workout and see how many calories you burn. During your first week stay with that number of calories. Each week increase the calories by an amount you can manage. You can also increase the time but don't go beyond 30 minutes. Combining more than 30 minutes of aerobics with 20 minutes of strength training nears the threshold beyond which making it a daily habit becomes difficult. The best is to stay at a maximum of 20 minutes aerobic and 20 minutes of strength training. Remember, a key to an effective exercise lifestyle is to never work so hard—or so long—that you don't want to come back the next day.

If you're walking or riding a bike for your aerobic exercise, the time limits remain the same. Ten to 20 minutes is ideal but don't go so long that you'll be discouraged from doing it every day. As your aerobic ability increases, you should attempt to increase the distance you go but not the time. Just as in working in a gym, once you get beyond 30 minutes, your ability to make that a lifestyle habit becomes more difficult.

Getting Started with Your Strength Workout

Many of you may never have done any strength workouts so we'll start with the most basic. Most strength workout programs deal with very specific muscles and muscle groups with terms like "delts" (deltoid muscles), "lats" (latissimus dorsi), "pecs" (pectoralis), "traps" (trapezius), "abs" (abdominal muscles), and many more muscles and muscle groups. The Type 2 Fitness Program simplifies all this by dividing your strength workout into three categories.

The three categories you'll work are very simply *your front, your core,* and *your back.* Using these categories dramatically simplifies the daily workout but still covers all the parts of your body needed for muscle enhancement, ratio of muscle to fat improvement, posture, and appearance improvement.

This is the program I've used for the past 15 years and it has served me very well. I have not done specific leg exercises but rather have counted on my eating and activity lifestyle to keep my legs in shape. More women than men seem to focus on adding strength workouts for their legs and that's simply a personal choice you can make. While women tend to gain weight on their legs and hips more commonly than men do, healthy eating combined with more activity will promote losing inches on hips and legs. Men are more prone to gain their weight on their bellies and often solve this problem by simply moving the front of their pants down inch by inch, year by year.

For women, doing leg exercises will make the muscles within your legs stronger and bigger but will not reduce the size of your legs or hips unless you combine it with the healthy eating and activity lifestyles you now know. For both men and women exercising "abs" will make those muscles stronger and bigger but it will not make your stomach slimmer or your waist smaller. What will make your stomach slimmer is combining your abs exercise with your new healthy eating and activity lifestyles.

The Importance of Eating More Protein

Before I outline the workout program, I'm going to talk once again about food—in this case protein. About 15 years ago, when I first began my workout program with my fitness trainer, Philip Bradfield, I noticed two other men working out as partners every morning at the same time. They appeared to be in their late 40s or early 50s. One was quite muscular with not much body fat. He was the workout leader of the two. The other man, the follower, was much less muscular with an average-looking body and a moderate amount of body fat.

For the full time Philip and I were in the gym for our sessions, these guys never talked to each other. They walked with purpose—sometimes bordering on what seemed like anger—from one machine to another. They alternated attacks on the machines. Grunting, pushing, yelling, and sweating. Generally working four or five times harder than I did during the time I was there. Every morning they were there driving themselves and each other with a passion that seemed to me to be impossible to sustain.

After a few months of noticing their intense daily workouts, I pulled Philip aside and said, "As hard as these guys are working, I haven't seen a bit of change in the follower, the guy with the average build." It was true. That guy had been killing himself for three months and nothing had changed.

Philip responded. "He's not eating right. His body has nothing to build with—no protein." He went on, "Usually people who work that hard and don't see results because they're not eating right, quit within the first month. He's lasted longer than most but he'll get discouraged and quit pretty soon when he realizes nothing's happening."

The message is this: If you want to see and feel results from your workouts, you need to increase the amount of protein you eat. Try to eat more eggs or egg whites, more fish, more chicken, pork, beef, steak, or hamburger. Some vegetables are also high in protein. As you develop your exercise program, you'll have more noticeable results if you eat more of these high-protein vegetables: spinach, peas, broccoli, and artichokes.

Remember that protein has very little impact on your blood sugar, and the vegetables I mentioned, even though they do have some carbohydrates, also have very little impact on your blood sugar. Eat more of these proteins and less of starchy carbs and sweet carbs, and you will gain muscle and lose fat with this program.

The Importance of "Front," "Core," and "Back" Workouts

Day one   works on the "front" part of your body (anterior shoulders, chest, and biceps). This muscle grouping is important for balance, strength, appearance, and increasing muscle-to-fat ratio.

Day two   works on the "core" part of your body (abdominal muscles, lower back muscles, and side muscles). This muscle grouping is very important in tying the upper part of your body to the lower part. They add athleticism and grace to movements and aid significantly in avoiding back problems for men and women. Men tend to have more back problems than women because with generally more upper body strength we tend to try and lift heavier objects. We're also generally a little taller, which puts more force on a lifting motion than a shorter person experiences. While women are certainly not immune to back problems, men can be divided into two categories: those who have back problems and those who will have back problems. Back problems can be diminished or avoided by strengthening core muscles.

Day three works on the "back" part of your body (upper back, triceps, and midback). This muscle grouping is usually the most ignored in many people's exercise programs. They are, however, very important for balance, erectness, and back health. Working only on the front muscles and ignoring the back results in a rolled-forward, slouching posture that is unhealthy and unattractive. Back workouts are a friend of good posture and good appearance.

Focusing each day on different parts of your body as I've described has three distinct advantages:

First, for those people who have not done any strength training this is very easy to categorize, and helps you remember where you are on any given day. For example, "Today is my day for 'front' or for 'core' or for 'back.'" You don't have to work so hard to recall the muscles worked on over the past few days.

Second, your muscles will get an automatic two-day rest between the times they are worked. Having at least one day for muscle rest and rebuilding is the one thing almost all strength-training gurus agree on. This program gives your muscles a two-day rest.

Third, the program works simply and beautifully with a three-day or six-day workout week.

The Patterns to Follow on All Three Days

All three workout days have the same pattern:

1. Start with a weight resistance that will allow you to do 25 to 30 repetitions. This will probably be a very light weight. This high number of repetitions is very important for people who have not exercised for a long time. You'll see I focus on the number of times (repetitions or reps) you should do and not the weight you should use. By focusing

on repetitions, you will automatically choose the appropriate weight for your level of strength.

2. The reason for the high number of repetitions is to allow your muscles to warm up. This warming up does two things.

3. First, it prevents injuries such as adhesive tendinitis, an irritation of the tendons which attach bone to muscle. If you don't start with very light resistance, you will feel tiny, almost imperceptible pops in the muscles you are working. These are little threads of tendons tearing. These micro tears won't hurt but they do cause a release of fluid that when it dries acts like super glue. Enough of these small tears will begin to restrict your range of motion to the extent that it will prevent your ability to reach behind your back or neck and even putting on a shirt or jacket can hurt.

4. Second, by warming up sufficiently you will be able to do subsequent repetitions with heavier weights and therefore better results.

5. Next, move to a heavier weight or resistance that allows you to do 20 repetitions. This is still a high number of repetitions so it should not be enough resistance to tear any tendons.

6. Finally, increase the weight or resistance to a level that will allow you to do 15 repetitions.

7. The weight or resistance you choose will be determined by the number of repetitions you are able to do. Obviously, your sets of 15 reps will be with a heavier weight than your sets of 20 and your sets of 20 will be with heavier weights than your sets of 25. You'll never need to increase those numbers but you will find with great satisfaction that within the first month you will naturally begin using heavier weights and more resistance for the same number of repetitions.

The Type 2 Workout Calendar

DAY ONE

Start with a 10- to 15-minute light aerobic workout described above followed by a "front" strength workout below.

Front (Anterior Muscles)

Biceps

25 reps with a starting weight of your choice

20 reps with a slightly heavier weight

15 reps with a heavier weight

Chest

25 reps with a starting weight of your choice

20 reps with a slightly heavier weight

15 reps with a heavier weight

Anterior Shoulders

25 reps with a starting weight of your choice

20 reps with a slightly heavier weight

15 reps with a heavier weight

You're done with your Day One strength workout.

AUTHOR'S NOTE:

Remember the weights are determined by your ability to do the number of reps that are called for. Your starting weight may be as light as five pounds or as heavy as 50 pounds or more. You may increase by increments as small as five pounds or as much as 20 or 30 pounds.

DAY TWO

Start with your aerobic workout followed by the "core" strength workout below.

Core

Abdominal Muscles (Abs)

(same pattern as day one)

25 reps with a starting weight or resistance of your choice

20 reps with a slightly heavier weight

15 reps with a heavier weight

Lower Back

25 reps with starting weight

20 reps with increased weight

15 reps with increased weight

AUTHOR'S NOTE:

This Day Two workout is just slightly longer than Day One or Day Three since it involves four muscle categories: Front, Lower Back, Left Side, and Right Side.

Sides
Left Side

25 reps with starting weight

20 reps with increased weight

15 reps with increased weight

Right Side

25 reps starting

20 reps increased weight

15 reps increased weight

You're now done with your "Day Two" strength workout.

DAY THREE

start with your aerobic workout followed by the "back" strength workout below.

Back (Posterior Muscles)

Triceps
(*same pattern*)
25 reps
20 reps
15 reps

Upper Back and Shoulders
25 reps
20 reps
15 reps

Mid-Back
25 reps
20 reps
15 reps

AUTHOR'S NOTE:

If you're doing this at home or anyplace you cannot adjust the weight, then just reverse the numerical sequence and it will have the same effect. For example start with 15 to warm up, then 20, then 25.

This Day Two workout is just slightly longer than Day One or Day Three since it involves four muscle categories: Front, Lower Back, Left Side, and Right Side.

You're now done with your Day Three strength workout.

If you choose to work out six days a week, repeat this pattern for Days Four, Five, and Six. Each muscle grouping will get two workouts in a week and two days of muscle rest before that group is worked again. Take the seventh day off and resume the pattern the following week.

If you choose to work out three days a week, simply repeat this pattern every other day with the seventh day off.

You'll find this simple pattern can become a habit and then a life-style. When you combine this exercise lifestyle with your new healthy eating lifestyle and more active lifestyle, you will lose weight, be healthier, feel stronger, look better, and generally enjoy your life more.

Getting Started

The descriptions of the machines to use and an explanation of the techniques for using them do not lend themselves well to a book like this one. The best thing to do is to go to a health club and ask for direction on using the machines. The danger there is that some young trainer may try to talk you into working harder and lifting heavier. Don't do it. Follow the pattern I've described.

Another option is to go online or pick up a book with photos of working different muscle groups. Just be sure to ignore all the advice about how hard you should work.

SECTION IV

Better Blood Sugar Control for Type 1 Diabetics and Insulin-Dependent Type 2 Diabetics

Chapter 12

Blood Sugar Testing for Good Control and Good Health

For insulin-dependent diabetics

Perfection is a dream. Excellence is attainable.
If you strive for excellence in all you do, once in a while perfection will appear.

—Rick Mystrom

Glucose Self-Testing— The Key to a Healthier Life for Diabetics

Though I've had diabetes for 50 years, self-testing has been available for only a little more than 30 years. The development of self-testing devices (blood glucose testers or meters; I'll call them "testers" from here on) is, in my opinion, the most important step in the potential improvement of diabetic health and quality of life since the discovery of insulin. I say "potential improvement," because the testers themselves are not going to make you healthier any more than buying a pair of walking shoes will make you healthier. You need to use your tester just as you need to use your walking shoes.

You don't need to test as often as I do but you do need to know when to test so that the results are meaningful. You need to know what to look for and how hat information will help your future decisions about eating. The glucose testers will also be instrumental in avoiding low blood sugars during normal daytime hours, during activities, and during your sleeping hours. Furthermore, testing will help in avoiding those foods that cause your blood sugar to rise too fast and too much. If you can learn that, your health and life will be much better.

How Close to Perfect Blood Sugar Control You Should Strive For

In chapter 2 I talked about the long-term consequences of high blood sugars, and in chapters 13 and 14 I cover in detail the immediate dangers of low blood sugars. To help you further understand balancing these two, I want to use an analogy that I started using in speeches a few years ago. This analogy is primarily for insulin-dependent diabetics, whether Type 1 or Type 2.

An Analogy to Illustrate the Risks and Rewards of Blood Sugar Control

Visualize yourself walking along on hard-packed ground. About six to 12 inches to your left is a six-foot drop-off to a sidewalk below. As you look ahead, you realize you have a long walk but you don't know how long. You can't even see your destination. It just disappears in a hazy horizon. But you know how important it is to get as far as you can and feel good striving for that destination. You also notice that the ground very near the drop-off on your left is dry and hard-packed and easy to walk on, but as you get farther away from the ledge, the ground becomes softer and muddier. The farther away from the drop-off, the softer and muddier the ground gets and the harder to walk on without wearing yourself out. You also notice that the transition from hard-packed, easy-to-walk-on ground to softer, muddier ground is gradual. So if you walk two feet away from the edge, the ground is a little softer than right along the edge and three feet out is still softer and harder to walk on; four and five feet out it is progressively softer and even harder to walk. Finally if you chose to walk six feet away from the ledge, you would have to struggle for every step and would be worn out very quickly.

Now you've got a choice. How close to the ledge do you walk? Well, your first reaction is, "That's simple. The first six to 12 inches nearest the ledge are absolutely dry, hard-packed, and easy walking, and the next foot away from the ledge is not too bad— just a little softer but still easy walking. I think I'll walk as close to the ledge as I can so I can go a long way without getting worn out."

That seems to make sense, but what if the journey is a long one—say, *the rest of your life?* Will you daydream a little and maybe step off the ledge? Will you make a misstep and fall off? Will you get dizzy and fall off? And if you do fall off, will you get hurt? It's not too far down—only about a six-foot drop. But you could get hurt. It's a sidewalk. You could even kill yourself if you landed wrong—unlikely, but possible.

So now let's bring that home to the issue at hand, diabetes. If you decide that you're going to shoot for perfect control, you're going to be walking along the ledge, less than a foot away from the drop-off for the rest of your life. To maintain perfect control of blood sugar levels through the use of insulin, you're going to risk some missteps in the form of periodic, serious low blood sugar episodes. These episodes are dangerous but not typically life-threatening, and they're certainly not fun and can cause injury. In my case, one caused a herniated disc.

If you're an insulin-dependent diabetic you may be making as many as 10 decisions a day on balancing food, exercise, and insulin. That's about 3,600 decisions a year. You're going to make some mistakes. I certainly have.

Now what happens if you choose the opposite path? You don't want to risk falling off the ledge so you choose to walk a long way away from the drop-off. In other words, you choose to not try for tight control but rather to let your blood sugars remain higher. After all, you don't necessarily feel bad immediately. You're a little tired but the degenerative consequences are not evident right away and you'll rarely, if ever, have a serious or extreme low blood sugar episode.

So what's the problem with that choice? Just like walking through that muddy, mucky ground, your body is going to wear out. You won't get very far. You'll be beset with complications. You won't live as long as someone who walks a little closer to the ledge.

So what's the right answer? For me the right answer has been to walk pretty close to the edge but not right on it. In other words, I didn't shoot for *perfection* in my blood sugar control but I shot for trying to be *very good* in my control (sort of halfway between perfect and good). If I were grading my blood sugar control, I'd give myself and A-minus for the past 30 years since self-testing first became available. For me though, the main reason for my health success is complementing my "less than perfect" control with a generally healthy eating, activity and exercise lifestyle.

Like most Type 1 diabetics, I'm going to see my blood sugar in the 300s a few times a month and in the 200s a couple of times a day. The important thing is that I correct those high blood sugars right away, using the adjustment factor that I discuss later in this chapter.

At 70 years old and in my 50th year as a diabetic and in excellent health, the balance between perfect blood sugars and good blood sugars has worked well for me. The result is I've been able to achieve long-term good health without letting diabetes dominate my life.

My Techniques for Testing My Blood Sugar

Earlier I told about how, during my first 16 years with diabetes, the results of a blood sugar test could take three days or more, so diabetics really couldn't determine how certain foods or exercise would affect their blood sugar. Maybe some diabetics went to a doctor every few months to have their blood drawn and sent to a lab for a blood sugar reading. If so, they would have a blood sugar reading about four times a year. For me it wasn't that often. For the first 10 years after I was diagnosed as a diabetic, I was moving a lot and didn't have a regular doctor. I don't recall having my blood sugar tested more than a half dozen times during that 10 year period—certainly less than once a year.

I moved to Alaska in my late 20s and began seeing a doctor regularly. Richard Witt was his name and I was happy with the relationship and conversations we had. I was busy with my family, my career, sports, and politics, so I met with Dr. Witt only a couple times a year for about six years. That meant only two blood sugar tests a year—a step up from the previous 10 years.

When I was 36, Dr. Witt retired and I was referred to Dr. Jeanne Bonar, with whom I've had a wonderful relationship for the past 34 years. About that same time, personal blood sugar testing became available. With encouragement and instruction from Dr. Bonar, I began testing my blood myself. The testing involved pricking my finger, blotting the blood on to a cardboard litmus strip and inserting it into a tester about the size of a paperback book. The whole process took about three or four minutes, but what a great improvement that was over the three days previously required.

Now the testers are much smaller and the process is much simpler and quicker. For me the process is about 15 seconds: five seconds to put a strip into the tester another five seconds to prick my finger and put the blood on the test strip and the final five seconds for the tester to give me a reading. So now instead of testing three or four times a year, I test between six and 10 times a day and often more.

I'll usually test five times a day if my blood sugar is in control and nothing out of the ordinary is happening and up to 10 or more times a day when my blood sugar is unexpectedly high or low, when I've eaten more than usual, when I've eaten atypical foods, or when I have a lot of activities going on. I've also learned to test before I give myself a shot just because I feel like my blood sugar is high. I used to count on what I felt my blood sugar was and give myself an infusion of insulin (called a bolus) but I got into trouble doing that when I thought it was high but was not.

The most common question I get when people see me testing or ask about testing is, "Does it hurt"? The answer is, "Yes, it hurts a little," but once I accepted testing as part of my life, it seemed to hurt less. It really comes back to keeping a positive attitude.

In testers, a lot of choices are available. Many testers offer weekly and monthly averaging and a recall feature that will show you hundreds of past tests and the ability to print them out on your or your doctor's computer. One of my close friends and neighbors on Finger Lake, Bob Niebrugge, has a tester that communicates directly to his pump. Another close friend, Al Bramstedt, just last week at Rotary showed me his continuous monitoring system that gave him real-time readouts of his blood sugar. It's not perfect at this time, as Al told me the following week. Readings are not yet consistently reliable but I'm sure they soon will be. The continuous monitoring system is very interesting to me and I expect I'll talk to Dr. Bonar about it in the future. But for now I'm happy with my separate testing and infusion.

While I understand the benefits of recall features to help communicate with your doctor, I've taken a different tack. Instead of having one tester that provides all those features, I've chosen to have a half dozen testers at different key locations in my daily life. I keep one tester in our master bedroom at our lake home, one in our bathroom, one in my home office, and one to put in my pocket when I leave the house. I also keep two in our townhouse in Anchorage. Using multiple testers as I do renders all the memory, data transfer, and print-out features relatively useless since the data are dispersed among six or more testers. However, I find by having testers conveniently located and easily accessible anywhere, anytime, I test more than I would if I used just one tester. Another advantage of my system that may be important to many folks is that the less technically sophisticated testers I use cost only about $20 each.

Make the "Basic Five" Daily Blood Sugar Tests Part of Your Daily Habit

The basic five daily blood sugar tests should be the core of your testing and will help you gain an understanding of the causes and effects of your blood sugar variations.

1. *Always test first thing in the morning.* This is your most important test. If your blood sugar is high, it has likely been so for eight hours or more. High blood sugar left unchecked for that length of time will contribute more to long-term problems than a high blood sugar for a shorter time. One of your most important goals is to wake up with blood sugars in your target range. My target range is 80 to 120. Waking up with a blood sugar less than 70 is a little dangerous. If your morning test is not what you want, try to figure out why that happened and how you'll try to correct it the next time.

2. *Test before lunch.* This test will tell you how well you did with your breakfast infusion (injection). In other words, did your insulin input match up well with the breakfast you ate? It will also give you your starting level for lunch. For me, if I find that I'm at 150 mg/dl before lunch, I give myself my best estimate for lunch plus one additional unit to compensate for the fact that my "before lunch" blood sugar was about 50 units high.

3. *Test before dinner.* This test is for the same reasons as above. It will tell you how you did with your lunch infusion and you'll know your starting blood sugar level prior to dinner. Follow the same adjustment process explained above for lunch.

4. *Test about one hour before bedtime.* The reason for this test is to establish a baseline and allow for any adjustment before you go to bed. Why is a baseline important? Let's say, for example, my blood sugar is 100 at this test. That's a very good number but it could also be a dangerous number if your blood sugar is going down and it could be an unhealthy number if your blood sugar is going up. This test, one hour before bedtime gives you a baseline for your bedtime test.

5. *Always test before bedtime.* Using the example from above in the test one hour before bedtime, let's look at three different possibilities. Your blood sugar is the same as in the previous test, your blood sugar is lower than in the previous test, or your blood sugar is higher than in the previous test. If it's the same as in the previous test, you can feel comfortable going to bed (or putting your child to bed) at that level. If it's lower, you need to take an appropriate number of glucose tablets or amount of sweet carbs. In this circumstance I would take a spoonful or two or three (depending on how much lower) of the Hershey's chocolate syrup I keep on my nightstand. (Then of course you'll need to rebrush your teeth). If this test is higher, you'll want to give yourself an appropriate infusion of insulin. ("Appropriate" means base it on your adjustment factor which I explain later in this chapter). I'm so confident of my adjustment factor and my pump's reliability that I can then go to sleep with no worry about low or high blood sugar during the night.

Know When You Should
Test Beyond the Basic Five Tests

1. *When you think your blood sugar may be low.* In this situation, do not put off or postpone testing. Test right away and if your blood sugar is low, assess the state of urgency associated with it. In the next three chapters I discuss the levels of urgency of different low blood sugar symptoms.

2. *When you eat an unusually big breakfast, lunch, or dinner* or have sweet or starchy carbohydrates at one of those meals. Then you should test midway between that meal and the next.

3. *When you're going into a situation where testing is highly inconvenient,* such as preparing to give a speech or conduct a meeting during which low blood sugar would affect your ability to think or speak lucidly.

4. *When you or your child are starting an activity that would likely lower blood sugar.* Good examples would be starting a hike, a run, a bike ride, a sport practice or competition, water sports, snow skiing, snow shoveling, cutting a lawn and so forth. For younger insulin-dependent diabetics those activities that necessitate a prior test would be any competition or play activity.

5. *When you feel your blood sugar is high and believe you may need an infusion of insulin.* This is pretty vague, but sometimes you may just feel like your blood sugar is high. Often it may have to be near 300 before you feel it but other times you may think it's high because you ate more than you

anticipated or infused too small an insulin dose. The key message here is *not* to give yourself an infusion of insulin just because you feel high. Make sure you're high before you infuse or inject the insulin. Always, always test before you give yourself a shot or an infusion in this situation. A few times I've given myself a shot or infusion when I just thought I was high and ended up with a serious or extreme low blood sugar reaction.

6. *When you've eaten fatty foods combined with starchy carbs for dinner and you've eaten a late dinner.* In this case you can expect your blood sugar to continue to rise while you're sleeping. You have a couple of options here. You can set a *temporary basal rate* that will increase your insulin going in for whatever number of hours you choose or you can use what's called a *square wave bolus*, which I learned about from my friend, Al Bramstadt, and had clarified by Kelly Foster, a medical professional. The square wave bolus puts insulin in at a slower rate for a longer period of time. This is ideal if you've eaten fatty foods for dinner. If you don't have enough confidence that you can hit the mark well enough with those features you might consider setting an alarm to wake up in a couple of hours and test again. Waking up at night to test sounds imposing but over the years, I've trained myself to wake up, test, adjust if necessary, and be back asleep in less than a minute.

7. *When you have a fairly large amount of insulin going in at bedtime.* For example, maybe I undershot on insulin for dinner and an hour before I'm going to sleep I test out at 300. I'll test again at bedtime. If it's still at that high level, I would give myself four units and that's a pretty big shot to be going in before I go to sleep. In this situation—which is

self- caused—I set an alarm so I can check again in a couple of hours and adjust if necessary.

8. You don't have to memorize all these situations—you just need to understand them and when one of them comes up you'll know it calls for an extra test.

Knowing Your Adjustment Factor— an Essential Part of Good Control

Every insulin-dependent diabetic, whether he or she uses a pump to infuse insulin or uses syringes to inject insulin, needs to learn *what his or her adjustment factor is.* Your adjustment factor very simply is how much one unit of insulin will reduce your blood sugar if all other factors are constant.

Why is that so important? Let's say in midafternoon I think my blood sugar may be high so I test my blood and find out it's 250. I sure don't want to leave it at 250; I want to bring it down to 100, which is the number I have used as a goal. (Some may use 90. Some may even use 80 but that's a little risky.) So to get my blood sugar down from 250 to 100, how much insulin do I give myself? By testing over the years, I've learned that my adjustment factor is 50. That means if I give myself one unit of insulin it will bring my blood sugar down 50 mg/dl. So here's the simple formula: 250 minus 100 (my goal) is 150. That means I have to bring my blood sugar down 150mg/dl. Since 150 divided by 50 (my adjustment factor) is 3, to bring my blood sugar from 250 down to 100 I'll give myself three units of insulin.

Very simple— but blood sugars don't always cooperate and are not always round numbers and not always as easy to divide and multiply as my example. Here's my shortcut: Let's say my blood sugar is 270. Subtract 100 and you obviously get 170. That's the amount I'd need to reduce my blood sugar by in this example. Instead of dividing that by 50, my adjustment factor, I divide it by 100 and get 1.7 and then multiply by 2 which equals 3.4. That's the amount of insulin I need to take to get my blood sugar down from 270 to 100. The logic behind my system is that it is much simpler to divide by 100 than it is to divide by 50. So dividing by 100 and then multiplying by 2 gives you the same result and it's very easy to do in my head.

It sounds a little convoluted but after doing it thousands of times, I can look at a number like 180 and say I need to give myself 1.6 units. Here's how I arrive at that: (180 minus 100 = 80, divided by 100 = .8 times 2 = 1.6 units). Let's say my test shows my blood sugar at 320. I know instantly that means a bolus (shot) of 4.4 units of insulin. Here's how I made that instant calculation: 320 minus 100 = 220, divided by 100 = 2.2 times 2 = 4.4 units. It takes me one or two seconds to make that calculation in my head (faster that I can punch it into a computer or calculator) and it will be the same for you after you've done it a few dozen times. This is the formula only if your adjustment factor is 50. If your adjustment factor is not 50, then you can create your own shortcut.

How do you arrive at your personal adjustment factor? It will take some experimenting and some time. Here's how to do it: Every time your blood sugar is a little high and fairly stable take your best guess as to how much insulin you'll need. Take your shot of insulin and then measure your blood sugar in two hours if you're using a pump or fast-acting insulin or three hours if you're using slower-acting insulin. Divide the drop in blood sugar by the number of units you injected or infused and the result will be your first rough idea of your adjustment factor. For example, if two units of insulin make your blood sugar go down 100 points, your adjustment factor is 50. If it takes four units of insulin to make your blood sugar go down 100 points, your adjustment factor is 25. Do this 10 or 20 times until you can predict within 10 points what your blood sugar will be. Now you've got your adjustment factor. You'll find it's a wonderful tool for blood sugar control.

Your adjustment factor could be anywhere from 10 points for a bigger person (meaning one unit of insulin would only lower your blood sugar 10 points) to 100 points for a smaller person (meaning one unit of insulin would lower your blood sugar by 100 points). Once you've determined it, follow my process above to derive your own shortcut using your own adjustment factor.

Here's the general formula:

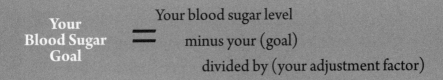

Your Blood Sugar Goal $=$ Your blood sugar level minus your (goal) divided by (your adjustment factor)

Example based on my adjustment factor of 50 and a blood sugar of 280
100mg/dl (my goal) =280 minus 100 = 180 divided by 50 = 3.6 units

Once you've mastered this concept your blood sugar control will be much easier and much better.

Adding the Judgment Factor to the Mathematics of Adjustment

If controlling your blood sugar was just pure mathematics, life would be simpler for insulin-dependent diabetics, but it's not just mathematics. It's also judgment. If my blood sugar is 250mg/dl and I want to get down to 100, it seems simple enough to subtract 100 (my target blood sugar) from 250 and then divide the difference (150) by my *adjustment factor* (50) and arrive at an appropriate insulin infusion of three units. That's the basic math of the formula and it's important to know how to apply it. However, other influences on your blood sugar also come into play.

1. *You may have food still being absorbed.* If you have eaten in the past two hours—longer if you've eaten some fatty foods—you'll need to add a little more insulin to your adjustment. How much additional insulin is something you'll learn over time.

2. *You may have insulin on board.* If you have insulin on board (going into your body), you'll need to reduce the amount of insulin your adjustment factor calls for. In this case it would be smart to test again within 30 to 45 minutes.

3. *You may be about to start a vigorous activity.* In this case you'll want to reduce the amount of the adjustment called for by your adjustment factor or maybe not adjust at all depending upon the intensity and length of the anticipated activity.

The Importance of Testing

Mary once said to me, "Which is more important, your insulin pump or your tester?" I hesitated for a moment and she jumped in. "I think it's your tester." I thought about her answer for just another moment and then agreed with her. I love my pump but if I hadn't had the ability to test easily, accurately, and conveniently for the past 30 years, I would not be healthy and likely not alive. I don't believe that overstates the value of testing.

By testing on a regular basis you will start learning about which foods in your eating patterns cause big rises in your blood sugar and therefore demand more insulin and contribute to weight gain, and which foods do the opposite. You have a great starting point in the chapters in this book on food but your own testing will confirm and personalize what you have learned there.

Whether you choose to have multiple testers as I do, or a single tester that can store and organize data is a personal decision determined by your lifestyle. Whatever your decision, do whatever you can to test as often as you can. The testers are cheap, but unfortunately the strips are very expensive. If you work for the federal government, your taxpayer-paid insurance program is the Cadillac of insurance programs and will pay pretty much for everything, including all the test strips you need. But if you work in the private sector you will probably have less coverage and greater deductibles. Even though you'll have to pay more than your federal counterparts, the money you pay for strips will be the best health investment you can make.

To insurance companies, here's my message: "If you don't pay for at least 150 to 200 test strips per month for your insulin-dependent customers, you're doing both your customers and yourselves a disservice. They will be less healthy and you will end up paying out much more in the long run to deal with the problems caused by insufficient blood testing."

Why You May Not Be a "Brittle Diabetic"

Over the past 30 years I've been a very high profile diabetic here in Alaska. As a consequence of that, I have a lot of diabetics come up to me with comments or questions about their diabetes. Some are knowledgeable about diabetes, some are not, some are positive and some are bitter. I offer advice and encouragement when asked and usually get good feedback.

One issue that concerns me, which comes up quite often, is when someone volunteers that he or she is a "brittle diabetic." Some will say they can't really control their blood sugar and their doctor said they were just brittle diabetics. Certainly they could have some thyroidal, adrenal, or psychological problems that may make their blood sugars erratic. But in my personal experience most just don't fully understand that every blood sugar level has a reason and an explanation. When I'm talking to a person who tells me he or she is a brittle diabetic, my first question is "Can you give me some examples of why you say that?" So far I've been able to explain every example of what these concerned diabetics see as an erratic, unexplainable blood sugar.

Here are two of the most common examples these diabetics, who have been told they're brittle, offer of unexplainably high blood sugars.

1. I'm a Brittle Diabetic Because
My Blood Sugar Rises Even if I Don't Eat Breakfast

Here's an example. One morning, a few years ago, an attractive and fit young woman (maybe in her early 20s) came up to me during my early-morning workout at the Alaska Club gym. She identified herself as a Type 1 diabetic like I was. Then she said, "But I'm a brittle diabetic." I said, "Why do you say that"? The first response she gave was, "That's what my doctor told me." I pressed further, "Can you give me some example of your brittle diabetes?" She said, "Yes. I just took my blood sugar five minutes ago and it's 300. When I woke up this morning it was about 110 and all I did was come into the gym and work out for almost an hour." She then repeated emphatically, "Now it's 300 and I didn't eat anything. How can that happen? I must be brittle." I asked if she had given herself a shot. "No," she said, "I didn't eat anything. Why would I give myself a shot?"

I explained to her that about 30 minutes before anyone wakes up in the morning, diabetic or not, their brain recognizes that they haven't eaten for eight or more hours and their cells need nourishment to prepare for normal morning activity. As they start the process of waking up, the liver starts to release some previously stored glycogen into the bloodstream. That glycogen turns to glucose in the bloodstream and provides energy to fuel the body until breakfast or until the next nourishment the body gets. That's part of the liver's function. If the cells aren't getting energy, the liver helps out by releasing stored glycogen. I continued, "For you as a Type 1 diabetic, your liver released the glycogen, which converts to glucose in your bloodstream, but your cells still couldn't get energy because your pancreas wouldn't produce insulin. Consequently, your blood sugar just kept going up." This morning process even has its own name, the "dawn syndrome."

Giving yourself a small shot in the morning even if you're not going to eat anything is one of the hardest things for an insulin-dependent diabetic to learn and do. It took me 10 years after I started testing to begin doing it on the rare occasion that I was not going to eat breakfast. Here' my advice for non-breakfast-eaters: I know it's hard to think about giving yourself a shot in the morning when your blood sugar is at the level you want and you're not planning on eating breakfast. Don't do it right away. For one week test your blood sugar one and two hours after you awaken and before you've eaten anything. I think you'll find blood sugars 150 to 200 points above what you woke up with. That's the "dawn syndrome." Once you've established your typical rise, then you can give yourself a small shot or bolus and be comfortable with the results.

2. And My Blood Sugar Goes Up Even When I'm Sleeping

The same girl listened very intently and when I finished she said, "Nobody ever told me that. It makes so much sense." She thanked me sincerely then said, "Does that happen at night too"? I said "No. Why?" She said, "Well, sometimes I measure my blood sugar before I go to bed and it may be 120 or so and I feel good about that. Then I may wake up two or three hours later because I'm feeling a little off— like my blood sugar is too high and I'll test to find out it is. It's sometimes in the 200s or even 300s. How can it go up when all I'm doing is sleeping?"

I asked her if she remembered what she ate for dinner when that happened and she said she didn't. I told her if she had any foods that contained a significant amount of fat plus starchy carbs for dinner, like steak or ribs with potatoes, rice, or bread, or maybe Mexican or Italian dishes, which generally include both fat and starchy carbs, the combination of fat and starchy carbs would explain her blood sugar rising at night. I explained that fat molecules are very stable and will take a longer time to break down and show up in her bloodstream. When fat is combined with starchy carbs it will cause a big rise in blood sugar that will continue for three or four hours.

I told her I was guessing that she had something like that for dinner on those nights she was talking about. I told her to pay attention to her dinners and see if they coincided with her blood sugar's rising while she was sleeping. I actually knew they would coincide but thought it would be more impactful if she came to that conclusion on her own.

She thanked me again. And although she didn't say it, I really feel that she will start to accept the fact that maybe she isn't a brittle diabetic. Maybe she'll discover all her blood sugars do have a reason and an explanation. She was a very interested listener and because she was so receptive, I can't help but think she took a major step toward better health that morning.

She was just one of maybe dozens of folks with whom I've had similar discussions. Maybe there are Type 1 diabetics who are brittle for some physiological or psychological reason. But I do believe that most who are diagnosed as brittle get that designation only because they, or their medical professionals, don't delve deeply enough into the logical cause and effect of their blood sugar changes. The downside for patients who may be designated as a brittle diabetic is that it gives them tacit permission to have high blood sugars. We all know now what the consequences of frequent and continual high blood sugars are.

My suggestion to those who have nighttime highs and think they may be brittle diabetics is to make a note of what you ate for dinner whenever you have nighttime highs. Then talk with your doctor about it. Even better, solve it yourself by eating a smaller mix of starchy carbs and fatty foods at dinner.

My own experience provides a pertinent example of what fatty foods will do if combined with starchy carbs for dinner. In the 1980s and early '90s, Mary and I and our kids would eat periodically at La Mex, our favorite Mexican restaurant in Anchorage. I would order a chili relleno and a cheese enchilada, which came with rice and refried beans, which I mostly did not finish. Often we didn't eat until seven or seven thirty, which is later than we now eat.

My typical infusion of insulin for dinner was about eight units. For that meal, which was bigger than most for me, I usually took 10 units. By bedtime my blood sugar would be pretty good, say 100 to 120, meaning that the amount of insulin I took balanced that meal fairly well *up to that point*. But I found that I'd then wake up in about three hours with blood sugar at 350 so. I'd take five more units of insulin and go back to sleep thinking that since every unit would bring my insulin down 50 points five units would get me down to 100. Not so. About two hours later, I'd wake up again and test. My blood sugar would still be around 300. I'd give myself four more units to try to bring my blood sugar down to 100. Finally when I woke up around 7 a.m., I'd test again and my blood sugar would be in the neighborhood of 100.

So what happened? Those were the days that I was eating more starchy carbs than I do now. The starchy carbs alone would cause a significant rise in my blood sugar and when mixed with slow-acting fat, the result was glucose entering into my bloodstream slowly but continuously for four or more hours. Because it went in slowly, my first infusion of 10 units brought my glucose down to the right level within two hours after I ate; but the mixture of starchy carbs and fat kept going in while I was sleeping and continued to raise my blood sugar.

Because that meal was larger than most of my dinners and it included significant amounts of starchy carbs and fat I typically ended up giving myself 19 or 20 units of insulin for a meal like that instead of my more typical eight to 10 units.

Here's the solution. If you like Mexican food, one option is to eat it for lunch. It will still go in slowly but that's exactly what you want when you still have 10 hours of activity before you'll go to bed. The bonus is that since the food will still be going into your bloodstream as glucose when you sit down for dinner, you won't feel as hungry at dinnertime. However, if you want to lose weight, one of the sacrifices you'll have to make is to cut back on Mexican foods.

If you do decide to have Mexican food for dinner, eat as early a dinner as possible and a smaller portion than you would usually have and try not to eat all the starchy carbs that come with the meal—especially rice, refried beans, and tortilla chips. Then try to be active for a while before you settle in for the evening. This pattern has worked well for me so I still get to enjoy the good food at La Mex once in a while.

Testing in Public Places

Maybe two or three years ago an advice columnist—I think it may have been Amy Dickenson, who writes the "Ask Amy" column in our newspaper, the *Anchorage Daily News*—received a question from a mother who had a diabetic daughter. The mother's question was this. "Our family was eating in a restaurant and before the food came I helped my daughter test her blood sugar. Some patrons sitting nearby were somewhat offended by this and said that we should have gone to the women's restroom to do that." "What do you think, Amy?"

Amy's answer was generally that the nearby patrons were right. Blood testing involving pricking a finger and getting blood should be done in a more private setting away from the other patrons—like a women's restroom in this case.

About two weeks later, Amy Dickenson—to her credit—headlined a retraction. She said she had never received so many responses disagreeing with any piece of advice she had given. She concluded that testing was so important and so necessary that there was no reason not to test right at a table in a restaurant.

I test in public all the time and I expect many of you do too. Don't be concerned at all about doing so. The more you test the more you'll learn and the healthier you'll be.

Conclusion

Testing is the window to your bloodstream. It's your teacher, your guide, your encourager. It reinforces correct actions you've taken and it reveals the results of incorrect actions. Every time your blood sugar is unexpectedly high, ask yourself what happened. Did you eat sweet carbs, too many starchy carbs, was it the dawn syndrome or did you eat too much fatty food for dinner? Every high blood sugar has a cause. The more you're able to determine what the cause of each one is, the better your control will become.

But don't forget the other more positive part of testing. When you hit 90 or 100 or 110 or whatever your target is, give yourself a pat on the back. It's a good feeling to have been right in your decisions. Enjoy it and smile.

Chapter 13

The Dangers of Too-Low Blood Sugars

For insulin-dependent diabetics

Some Things to Recall As You Begin This Chapter

Almost all foods are converted to some amount of glucose as they are absorbed through the stomach lining and into the bloodstream. Some foods create a lot of glucose (sugar) in your bloodstream. Other foods create less glucose. Some foods enter your bloodstream as glucose very quickly. Other foods enter more slowly. These factors are important to understand.

AUTHOR'S NOTE:

Because of the importance of this chapter parts of it also appeared in my first book, My Wonderful Life with Diabetes.

The other issue to be aware of is that your brain needs a minimum amount of glucose to function. If your glucose gets below a certain level, your brain cannot function properly and if your glucose gets extremely low, you cannot maintain consciousness and may have a seizure.

Low Blood Sugars and Their Consequences

One diabetic control issue that I did not handle as well as I could have during my first 30 years as a diabetic is avoidance of extreme low blood sugars. During those first 30 years with diabetes I experienced nine low blood sugar episodes that required trips to hospital emergency rooms, though only one that I recall required an overnight stay at a hospital.

About half of my "extreme" low blood sugar episodes occurred in the 16 years before self-testing. Almost every case was carelessness and/or lack of knowledge on my part, or what can honestly be called pilot error. The rest occurred after self-testing was available. But after about 10 years with self-testing I figured things out and have not had a low blood sugar seizure in the past 20 years.

According to Dr. Bonar, who has had thousands of diabetic patients over the past 40 years through her large practice, my nine extreme low blood sugar episodes in 50 years is actually better than most. She is especially pleased that in the past 20 years I have experienced zero episodes requiring emergency help or trips to an emergency room. Nine episodes in my first 30 years as a diabetic was an average of one every three and one third years. In my opinion, that's too many, especially with current technology. However, Dr. Bonar told me that many newer, younger Type 1 diabetics may have one a year or more. Some of the more careless new diabetics may have multiple trips to an emergency room in a single month.

As you learned in the previous chapter, the number of low blood sugar episodes requiring emergency help is also determined by how close to perfection your blood sugar goals are. The closer you strive to perfection, the more potentially low blood sugars you are likely to have and the more vigilance you'll need.

Since I haven't had an extreme low blood sugar episode in 20 years, that's brought my average number of episodes per year down to less than one every five years or so. Better—but not as good as your record can be by following the advice in this book. It took me over 30 years to learn how to keep good control and still avoid these frightening and traumatic experiences. In just a few hours with this book, you can learn what it took me over 30 years to learn.

People often ask "What does low blood sugar feel like?" My simple and short explanation goes something like this. My first indication of low blood sugar is feeling a little shaky and nervous. Not unlike the feelings I used to have before starting a hurdles race in high school or getting up before my speech class in college.

If my blood sugar continues down, the next symptom is confusion. My brain becomes short on the nutrients needed to connect thoughts. If my blood sugar is very low, I will sometimes stand in front of an open refrigerator door looking at the orange juice or Coke I need to raise my blood sugar but not able to think clearly enough to reach in and get the very thing I need.

A good description of the degrees of hypoglycemia (low blood sugar) is given in the book, *The Johns Hopkins Guide to Diabetes*[1]. The authors divide hypoglycemia into three stages:

Mild Hypoglycemia	When you are mildly hypoglycemic, the symptoms are mainly physical: sweating, trembling, and so on. You can recognize them. You may notice that you aren't thinking as clearly as you usually do or that you aren't behaving quite normally, though others might not notice these subtle changes.
	Even mild hypoglycemia can be distressing, but most people don't find these episodes terribly upsetting.

1   Saudek, Christopher D., M.D.; Rubin, Richard R., Ph.D., CDE; Shump, R.N., CDE. (1997). *The Johns Hopkins Guide to Diabetes for Today and Tomorrow*; Baltimore and London, Johns Hopkins University Press.

Moderate Hypoglycemia	When you are moderately hypoglycemic, you may become confused or act inappropriately, but you can still treat the low blood sugar yourself.

Severe Hypoglycemia	When you are severely hypoglycemic, you are no longer able to self-treat. You may even fall into a coma or suffer a seizure.

For purposes of my book, I split up *severe hypoglycemia*. I continue to use that term to describe being unable to put your thoughts together to self-treat and needing someone else to help to get some form of sugar into your system. But I remove reference to a seizure or coma from that category and add a fourth category: *Extreme hypoglycemia*.

Extreme Hypoglycemia	When you are extremely hypoglycemic you may suffer a seizure and require professional emergency help (paramedics or fire department) and/or transportation to an emergency facility.

I'll use these terms throughout this section to describe the stages of hypoglycemia (low blood sugar). Additional factors must also be considered. For example, moderate hypoglycemia with insulin and no food going into your system can become severe hypoglycemia very quickly. But moderate hypoglycemia with food going into your system faster than insulin is going in is not a problem. It's also important to note that throughout this book I'll use the terms *hypoglycemic reaction* and *low blood sugar reaction* interchangeably.

By applying what you learn in this book you will be able to minimize or completely avoid these reactions.

Symptoms of Low Blood Sugar by the Numbers

In the United States, blood sugar is measured by the term *mg/dl*, which is milligrams of glucose per deciliter of blood. So when you measure your blood sugar using any one of the scores of testers available, the number on your device is telling you the *milligrams of glucose per deciliter* of your blood at that moment.

Many testers have a history function and an averaging function, which can be very helpful in demonstrating your progress in keeping your blood sugars under control. As I've noted previously, those functions are not particularly useful for me because I choose to use multiple testers. So the personal decision for you is whether to just use one tester and gain the benefit of your blood sugar history, or use multiple testers and gain the benefit of convenience for frequent testing.

For insulin-dependent diabetics or those with loved ones who are insulin-dependent diabetics, I've created a more detailed explanation of the symptoms of low blood sugar by the numbers. Below are the low blood sugar symptoms that I've experienced at different levels over the past 30 years of self-testing. As you read these levels you will notice some overlap. For example, 70mg/dl could fit in the first category or the second category. This overlap is simply because this is not intended to imply a specificity that cannot be felt. These are intended to be general categories and may differ slightly between different people.

110 mg/dl down to 70 mg/dl

These are ideal levels. Everything feels fine. I can think clearly. My coordination is good. I sleep well. I can hit a golf ball straight, though normal blood sugar doesn't guarantee that I always will.

70 down to 60

I can begin to feel these lows. I notice weakness when I'm doing anything strenuous like climbing hills or stairs, lifting, shoveling snow, playing tennis and so on. When I'm not doing anything strenuous, I may not feel anything abnormal. In this range I begin to experience a little loss of eye-hand coordination, which will manifest itself in erratic golf shots.

It's also important to note that doing something very intense or competitive may mask symptoms at these or even lower levels. Water-skiing is a good example. When waterskiing, I'm often focused, intense, and in very cold water. All those factors cause a drop in blood sugar levels. A number of times while waterskiing, I've got down to 50 without feeling it. One time, which you will read about in the next chapter, "Avoiding Dangerous Lows," waterskiing resulted in an extreme low blood sugar, which led to unconsciousness and an ambulance trip to a hospital emergency room in Hot Springs, Arkansas.

60 down to 55

This is the level where I will feel weak even if I'm totally sedentary: reading, talking, watching TV and such. I feel less energetic and as my kids would say, a little irritable. This level alone is not dangerous, but the important issue at this level is how fast your blood sugar is going down. If you don't have much insulin on board, in other words, going into your body, this level is not an emergency situation, but if you do have insulin on board and no food going in, this requires quick action.

55 down to 50

At this level I have difficulty completing complex thoughts. I'll get partway through explaining a thought and be unable to finish it. At that point I'll often stop and tell whoever I'm conversing with that my blood sugar is low and I need something with sugar--soft drink, candy, apple juice, orange juice and so forth.

The other symptom at this level is a significant loss of motor skills. This is most obvious for me in the sport of golf. Other sports that require hand-eye coordination but not such detailed precision don't typically alert me to a low blood sugar problem as quickly as golf does.

I can recall times on the driving range when I was hitting the ball just fine, then out of nowhere I'll start miss-hitting balls—five, six, seven in a row—before it occurs to me to measure my blood sugar. I measure and most of the time find that my blood sugar is in the 50–55 range.

When I'm playing golf, low blood sugars in this range manifest themselves with three or four terrible miss-hits in a row. Now I'm perfectly capable of two or three bad shots on a hole even if my blood sugar is normal so that's not always a reliable indicator.

50 down to 45

At this level of low blood sugar, I can't read a magazine, newspaper, or a book. The pages appear to have bright spots all over them that mask many of the words. I also begin to see bright flashes around the room I'm in. I quickly realize what the problem is and what the solution is. I know I have to get something into my body as quickly as I can to raise my blood sugar. At this level, I can still figure out what I have to do and do it. I can solve things myself as long as Coke, juice, or Skittles are handy.

45 down to 40

At this blood sugar level it's very difficult for me to help myself. I know something is wrong but I can't always figure out what is happening. My decision making is impaired. This is an urgent problem. Even when I figure out that I need something from the refrigerator, a number of times I've gone into the kitchen, opened the door to the refrigerator, and stood there in front of the open door and just stared in not knowing what to do.

At this level it's essential to call out to someone for help. For me it's usually my wife, Mary, who will quickly mix chocolate syrup with coke and hand it to me. By that time I'm usually sitting on the floor or on a step with my head in my hands. The chocolate in the Coke makes the Coke flatter and easier to drink quickly. And quick is essential. At that point I don't worry about putting too much sugar in my body because the consequences of my blood sugar continuing down are so much more serious than the consequences of my blood sugar going up too much.

The confusion that results from this level and below is the very reason that it is so important that family and friends know what to do and how to help. They need to ask, "Are you okay?" "Do you need some sugar, a soft drink, or a candy bar?" Most of the time you'll have solved this problem before it gets to this stage. You will have felt your sugar getting lower and eaten or drunk something to raise your blood sugar, but if you haven't caught it in time, you need to count on your family or friends.

Even in a public place you need to ask someone for help before you get so confused you can't ask. I recall one time during my second term as mayor, I was driving in to City Hall and realized my blood sugar level was dangerously low and I needed something quickly. The City Market was on my route just a few blocks ahead. When I reached it I turned a hard left, parked my car, and walked quickly into the market. By that time, though, I was beyond the point of being able to find any soft drinks or help myself in any way. I stood near the entrance holding on to the edge of a display rack. The next person to walk in was a lady who stopped, put her hand on my arm and said, "Are you okay?" "No," I said. "I need some sugar quick." She grabbed a Pepsi off a shelf about ten steps away, opened it and had it in my hand in no time. Within two minutes or so my blood sugar had gone up enough for me to realize the crisis had passed. I thanked her but never got her name. So whoever you are, thank you again for realizing I needed help and helping.

A second episode requiring me to ask for help publicly happened at the Ryder Cup Golf Match at the Medinah Golf Club near Chicago in October 2012. I had traveled from Alaska to Chicago with 13 Alaskan friends to see the matches featuring the best American golfers vs. the best European golfers and to play some golf ourselves.

During the first day of the three-day contest, I had been watching the matches with three of my friends, Eldon Mulder, James Armstrong, and Craig Tillery. We had been moving around the course and watching the contest from various locations. By the end of the day we had been walking and standing for about 10 hours. That in itself is not a big deal, but the significance is that continual movement such as that for so many hours burns a lot of calories and brings down blood sugar much faster and more consistently that a normal day's activity for me. I'd had only a hot dog with half the bun for lunch with a bottle of water to drink—not much in the way of calories or blood sugar support for the activity that day.

About 4 p.m. I could feel my blood sugar getting low but that wasn't a problem, since I had a regular-size packet of M&Ms in my pocket along with my omnipresent Halloween-size packet of Skittles. I ate the full packet of M&Ms and felt confident that would bring my blood sugar up sufficiently until we stopped for dinner on the way back to the house where we were staying.

As that day's matches ended at about 6 p.m., we began making our way with thousands of other spectators toward the busses which would take us to the Arlington Race Track, where all the cars were parked. As we had just exited the golf course my blood sugar felt low again. I shouted to my friends to wait because I was going to test my blood sugar. It was 45 and likely going down since I was continuously burning calories and using glucose in my blood. But I still had my small packet of Skittles. I popped those in my mouth in hopes it would stop the drop in blood sugar as it almost always did. This time, however, it wasn't enough. The glucose I was burning overrode the input of sugar from the Skittles and by the time I got on the bus, my blood sugar was 40.

I knew my blood sugar was still going down because of the continuation effect of exercise. Blood sugar will typically continue down for up to a half hour after exercise or activity is complete. Eldon had thoughtfully asked for a quick primer on what to do if I lost consciousness. I told him to just try to keep me from hurting myself and have someone call 911. Then I stood up in the darkened bus and announced that I had diabetes and needed something sweet right away. A man a few seats in front of me had a half full bottle of Sprite, someone else passed me some Lifesavers and a woman's voice behind me asked if pretzels would help. "They will," I said.

I drank the remaining Sprite, ate the Lifesavers, and had some of the pretzels. Within minutes my blood sugar was up and everything was back to normal. It can be tough to do but sometimes you may need to ask for help publicly. Do it without hesitation. People will help.

40 down to 30

This is serious and urgent. If you have insulin going in you may be a minute or two from seizure and unconsciousness. You don't have time to measure your blood sugar. You just have to know the symptoms: confusion, brightness to the point you can't see well, inability to recognize your surroundings. At this level I can't find the refrigerator; I can't find a door to get out of or into my house, I can't find a soft drink or candy in a grocery store, and I've been unable to find the door of a convenience store even as I stood in its parking lot.

You must understand the urgency at this blood sugar level. Don't wait. Act immediately. Call to anyone nearby to help you. Although I haven't had any extreme low blood sugars requiring medical help in the past 20 years, I have had a couple of close calls with my blood sugar below 40.

On an early summer morning a year ago, I woke up realizing my blood sugar was dangerously low. Based on the symptoms it was probably below 40. I walked out to the living room and shouted for Mary. But she was outside watering her flowers. It's a common early-morning enjoyment of hers and somehow I remembered that, but I couldn't find the door to get out to where I knew she was. This is a house that has seven doors leading outside and I couldn't find one. My brain was starved for glucose and was shorting out.

Everything was bright and confusing. I couldn't find the refrigerator. I stumbled across the door leading out to the garage and saw an unopened twelve-pack of Cokes in a cardboard container. I tried to figure out how to open the box along the perforated lines but couldn't. A coke was exactly what I needed but I couldn't think clearly enough to just rip open the box.

I wandered back into the living room and yelled again for Mary. No answer. I straggled into our bathroom—nothing there. Then I wandered into our bedroom, where I had started four or five minutes before. There on my nightstand was a Coke and some chocolate syrup. I sat on my bed weak and confused and alternated sips of Coke with the chocolate.

In a matter of minutes my blood sugar started to come back up. Within three or four minutes my blood sugar was high enough for me to walk into the living room, out the 12-foot-high doors that lead outside to the flowers on the south patio, and tell Mary what had happened. Walking out the door to get help sounds so simple but it's not when your blood sugar is so low that your brain can't function. You can look right at a door and still not see it.

If you catch the low blood sugar in time, as I did in this instance, you'll feel absolutely normal in a matter of minutes with no repercussions. If you don't catch it in time, you're in for a seizure, unconsciousness, and an ambulance ride to the hospital. And that's no fun. Not to mention the possibility of injury caused by falling (usually face first) during a seizure.

Below 30

Only once have I been below 30 and still been conscious. That was about 20 years ago, when I recall registering a 27 on my glucose meter. Hopefully you (or your diabetic child or loved one) will never get that low or lower but if you do, it's important to know what to expect.

If you as an insulin-dependent diabetic have your blood sugar drop into the 30s and have insulin on board but no food going in, you are likely going to continue down until you get into the 20s and you will have a seizure and lose consciousness. From that point on you will be aware of nothing. No pain. No time awareness. No dreams. No memory. Nothing. It's much like being under anesthesia without medical supervision and with a seizure thrown in.

My experience with emergency medical technicians is that they are well trained in dealing with extreme low blood sugar situations. According to my wife, the first thing they do is test my blood sugar. They then put in an IV (intravenous drip) of what's colloquially called DW50. That's 50 percent dextrose and 50 percent water. That begins the process of bringing my blood sugar up.

Usually I don't begin to gain any awareness until I'm in the emergency room at a hospital. However, twice in longer ambulance rides I became semiconscious in the ambulance. In the emergency room I gradually become aware of people around me talking about me. Almost always the very first thing I remember is a doctor or a nurse saying "He's starting to come around." My blood sugar starts approaching normal levels and things start to clear up very quickly for me. Within about 15 minutes I start having conversations with the doctor or nurse and within half an hour I'm ready to leave.

Twice I recall being injured in an extreme low blood sugar episode. Once I fell face first on the tile floor of a McDonald's restaurant and ended up with a black eye and a bruised nose. A second time my convulsions were so extreme that I herniated a disc in my back which required an operation—successful, I'm pleased to report. That operation was in 1991 and I haven't had a back problem since.

What if No Emergency Help Is Available

Periodically someone will ask me what happens if no medical help or other help is available. If you're on your own and unconscious, then what happens? I've had only one experience with that situation. I was at the Golden Horn Lodge, a fishing lodge in western Alaska, run at the time by my friends, Bud and Holly Hobson. I was fishing the first day with Doug Dicken, a board member of my advertising agency, and my eight-year-old son, Rich. Rich and I were bunking together. Sometime during that night my blood sugar had gone below the level that would allow me to remain conscious. I woke up about 5 a.m. on the floor with sore muscles, bruised elbows, and a knot on my head. I had experienced an extreme low blood sugar episode during the night, but came back to consciousness without outside help.

What I have since learned is that convulsions trigger the release of adrenaline, which in turn releases glycogen (a version of glucose) from the liver. So even if you're out in the woods, the backcountry or alone anywhere and you have a convulsion and lose consciousness, you will likely recover naturally. The danger of course is injury to yourself and/or exposure to the elements.

Extreme low blood sugar episodes are not to be taken lightly. They're emotionally draining. They can be dangerous. And they scare the heck out of family members. So my advice to you is, "Don't let this happen to you." It took me almost 30 years to figure out the keys to avoidance. You can learn them in 30 minutes in the next chapter.

Chapter 14

Avoiding Extreme
Low Blood Sugar Episodes

Very important for Type 1 or Type 2 insulin-dependent diabetics

Too Many Extreme Low Blood Sugar Episodes

I assign very little blame for the frequency of my extreme low blood sugar episodes to my attempts to keep my blood sugar in tight control. I assign much more blame to my lack of understanding the simple steps to avoiding these serious lows. When I add in a combination of carelessness, distraction, and probably a hint of feeling invulnerable as a young man, I've got a pretty good recipe for having too many extreme low blood sugar episodes.

It's taken me a long time to really understand how to avoid these extreme low blood sugars. Now I understand what it takes and what habits every insulin-dependent diabetic needs to develop in order to avoid these episodes. By applying this information, I have not had an extreme low blood sugar reaction for about 20 years—by far the longest period of emergency-free low blood sugar episodes in my diabetic life.

One of the greatest benefits that an insulin-dependent diabetic will get from reading this book is an understanding of the actions to avoid extreme low blood sugar episodes. This means understanding how you should react to low blood sugars based on *three categories of urgency* and understanding the *six steps to avoid low blood sugars* at the end of this chapter. I've chosen to summarize these steps and actions required after I relate to the readers the results and causes of my personal episodes.

Understanding My Personal Emergency Experiences Will Help You Avoid Them

In my companion book, *My Wonderful Life with Diabetes*, I've told the stories of five extreme low blood sugar episodes I had in the 1970s before the advent of personal blood sugar testing. In those cases I really didn't know exactly what the causes were. After testing became available in the early 1980s, I began to understand the specifics of why these episodes were happening and what mistakes I had made to cause them. Self-testing certainly doesn't eliminate the possibility of extreme low blood sugar episodes, but it does give you the tools to dramatically reduce the possibility of them.

What is it that I've learned about keeping good control, being active, and staying healthy, yet not having any blood sugar episodes requiring emergency treatment?

In this chapter, I'll explain how these extreme low blood sugars happened to me and what mistakes I made to cause them. By reading about my experiences and their causes, you will begin to understand how and why they happened to me and how you can avoid them. I'll conclude this chapter with the steps you can take to avoid these distressing, disrupting, and potentially dangerous experiences.

Extreme Low Blood Sugar Episodes and the Mistakes That Caused Them

Lake Ouachita near Hot Springs, Arkansas 1983

Our family was in the southeast United States on one of our family vacations. We had stopped in Memphis to visit Dave and Skippy Morton and their family, with whom I had spent many weekends throughout my college years. We then traveled west to Arkansas to visit their oldest son and my closest friend, Asa. Another close friend of ours from college days, Steve Kinney, flew in from Colorado to join us.

Asa had started a company called American Interplex in Little Rock, Arkansas and was starting to accumulate a little discretionary income. He had purchased a small waterski boat and was anxious to take us waterskiing. Though it was late spring with an air temperature of about 60 degrees and the water temperature about the same, our family was willing and ready to go, though we were brand-new to waterskiing. "As usual, the Mystrom family was ready to try anything," is the way Asa put it.

We rented a couple of small cabins on the lake for a few days of waterskiing. Asa was patient with all of us as we finally mastered getting up on two skis, then staying up just long enough to get comfortable before dropping one ski in our beginning attempts to slalom.

By the second day we were all waterskiing much better, but the cold water and air made for a midafternoon finish. By the time we were ready to call it a day, we were cold, wet, and tired but we had had a great time. This was my first lesson on how fast being both cold and active, especially in the water, can consume calories and lower one's blood sugar.

By that stage in my diabetic understanding I was very aware that activity adds to the effect of insulin so that insulin plus activity will lower blood sugar faster than just insulin alone. What I was not aware of was how being in cold water adds dramatically to the calorie-burning and blood–sugar-lowering impact of an activity. Calories are a measure of heat, and the greater the heat differential between your body at 98.6 degrees and your surroundings (in this case 60-degree water) the more calories you will burn, and the faster your blood sugar will drop. With the intense activity of waterskiing and the calorie-burning water temperature, I shouldn't have gotten in the water to ski with my blood sugar less than 200 or so.

Three factors I should have considered before I started this activity. First was my blood sugar level when we started the activity. Second was how much insulin I had on board when we started. The final factor coming into play is what I call the "unusual activity" factor. A danger arises when you're engaged in an activity that you're generally unfamiliar with. You tend to be focused very intently on the activity and you are not as sensitive as you should be to what's happening to your blood sugar. You may not feel the low until it's too late.

In any case, my decisions weren't correct. As Asa pulled in to dock the boat, I stepped off to tie it up. For the first time, I noticed that my blood sugar felt low. Amazingly, I didn't have my tester or any emergency sweets or glucose tablets handy (just one more mistake in the sequence) but a store was just about 200 yards from the dock. I started walking toward the store. I don't recall if I asked Steve to join me or if he just came along. We got to the store. I recall stepping in and starting to tear some wrapping off a candy bar. That was the last thing that I recall.

Recalling the incident nearly 30 years later, Steve said I didn't mention anything about my blood sugar being low. His recollection was that I took a candy bar off the counter and started eating it right there. He paid for it, then we walked out of the store. We had walked about 50 yards back toward the dock when I became unresponsive. According to Steve, "Your eyes rolled back in your head."

In this instance I had already started eating a candy bar, which would usually enter my bloodstream within two to three minutes. But it was too late and too little. My blood sugar had dropped to a level that wouldn't sustain consciousness before the sugar from the candy reached my bloodstream.

According to Mary, Steve ran back to the cabin yelling that I needed some insulin—exactly what I didn't need. Mary knew that, of course. But it's a very common misperception that if a diabetic is confused or unconscious, insulin is needed. In fact, in almost all cases the opposite is true. I tell people that it's always safe to try to get something sweet into a diabetic who appears to be confused or unresponsive. That condition is almost always caused by low blood sugar, not by high blood sugar. In the remote case that it is caused by high blood sugar, additional sugar is not going to help but it is also not going to be a dangerous short-term action.

Asa's recollection was that Steve came running to the dock "yelling at the top of his lungs that Rick needed help."

In asking each of the three to search their memories for the details of this event 30 years ago, each story was slightly different. So when I asked what happened after I collapsed in the parking lot, Steve's reaction was, "We couldn't move you so I went up to the porch of the cabin to have a cigarette and wait for the ambulance." I said, "Steve, you mean you left me lying on the parking lot while you went to the porch to have a cigarette?" He said, "Yeah, but I could see you and you looked comfortable." Mary's story reflects a little more compassion and I prefer her description of lovingly stroking my head as I lay there.

I started to regain consciousness in the ambulance on the way to the Hot Springs hospital even though the medics did not administer dextrose and water. Within about 30 minutes after the doctor at the emergency room started an intravenous solution of dextrose and water, I recovered and started feeling okay. We were all hungry after this episode so we went to a pancake house to eat and talk about how lucky it was that it didn't happen when I was in the water.

In this instance as in most, I was out of the hospital and feeling fine within an hour or so with no repercussions. But it doesn't always happen that way. In the next example, I got a little beat up.

Mistakes That Caused This Episode

1. Not being aware of what my blood sugar level was at the start of the activity

2. Not understanding the compounding impact of strenuous activity plus being in cold water

3. Not having emergency glucose or candy in the boat

4. Not measuring my blood sugar during the activity

As you can see, it was a combination of mistakes on my part. More often than not it's multiple mistakes that have caused my unconsciousness. One mistake can often be corrected and problems avoided by doing other things correctly. In this case, mistakes one and two would not have resulted in hospitalization if I had just measured my blood sugar more often or had some form of sweets or sugared drink on board the boat.

McDonald's in Anchorage 1984

It was a sunny spring day in Anchorage. The snow had melted, the roads were dry. It was the kind of day that made me think, "If I get my car washed today, it may stay clean for a week." I was in my fairly new and very dirty BMW in line at the neighborhood car wash with a few cars in front and another dozen behind me.

About the time I got to the front of the line and felt my car move forward slightly as it firmly connected to the automatic track system that would pull my car through the car wash, I sensed my blood sugar was low. I also remembered that I had given myself an infusion of insulin about 30 minutes before, thinking I would stop and get a hamburger someplace. But I got sidetracked and had still not eaten anything.

Still, this was nothing urgent or problematic, I thought, as long as I could have some soda, juice, or candy within five minutes or so.

I looked in the glove box of my car. Nothing I could eat in there but lip balm and I was pretty sure there were no calories in that. There were cars ahead of me and behind me and because the car wash was so crowded, everything was moving more slowly than usual. By the time I got out of the car wash my blood sugar was so low that I couldn't make good decisions or think in a logical, linear process (I'm guessing it was in the neighborhood of 40 to 45 mg/dl). Had I been able to think with any clarity, I would have realized that I could have gotten a candy bar or a soda right across the street at the Carr's grocery store. But I couldn't figure that out.

I pulled out onto the street and couldn't figure out which way to go. Somehow I remembered McDonald's, about a mile away. I had driven past it thousands of times in the past 12 years, but now everything seemed very bright and I didn't recognize any stores or signs as I drove.

I conjured up every ounce of concentration I could to try to figure out where I was. Then I saw the unmistakable McDonald's arch at the corner of Northern Lights and Arctic Boulevards. I pulled into the parking lot, walked into the restaurant and then in one of the stupidest, deferential moments of my life, *I got in line.* Clearly, in retrospect, I should have gone right up to the counter and told a clerk, "I'm a diabetic and I need a coke right now."

I didn't do that. I got in line. That's the last thing I remember before I started coming to in the emergency room at Providence Hospital. Everything seemed foggy. I could hear people talking about me. Then I could make out people in white smocks, some with simple cloth hats on their heads. Then I heard the words, "He's coming around." "Rick, how are you feeling?" My nose hurt. My forehead and one eye socket hurt. An IV was attached to the back of my hand. But things were coming into focus. Within 15 minutes I was talking to the doctors and nurses and we all knew I was going to be fine.

I stayed in the hospital until that evening because I was pretty banged up. I had fallen face first on the tile floor at McDonald's and had a swollen nose, black eye, and a pretty good sized bump on my forehead.

Mary was at the hospital right away, as was Dr. Bonar. Bill Pargeter, the owner of the McDonald's franchises in Alaska, showed up within an hour. Not only was Bill a client of Mystrom Advertising, but he was also a friend. He was very aware of what had happened since his daughter had Type 1 diabetes too.

Linda Boochever, the vice president of my company, was also there. I overheard her talking to one of our employees back at the office. Whoever she was talking to must have asked if I was okay. All I overheard was, "No, he's not okay."

I was back in the office the next day. I remember missing that afternoon at work was a big deal to me because in the 20 or so years I had been working up to that time, I had never taken a sick day.

As in all my extreme low blood sugar reactions, from the time I lost consciousness to the time I woke up in the emergency room everything was a blank. No memories. No pain. No awareness of the passage of time. No dreams. Nothing. I used to describe it as being dead for a couple of hours but a friend used the analogy of being under anesthesia and I think that's a better comparison.

Mistakes That Caused This Episode

1. Giving myself a shot too far in advance of my eating.

2. This is an issue that some may disagree with me on. Some may say it's better to give yourself a shot half hour or so in advance of eating. There are good arguments for that tactic. It gives the insulin a chance to begin absorbing into your body before you eat and can compensate for the fact that some of the food you may typically eat at a meal will get

into your bloodstream faster than the insulin will. So in a sense it gives the insulin a head start over the food and will prevent a short-term rise in your blood sugar as you're eating. That makes sense, but the downside side is just what happened to me. You can't delay or forget eating once you've taken your shot. So it's a judgment call, but now I choose to wait until I have the food in front of me. I know I'm going to eat and I know exactly what I'm going to eat, which makes it easy for me to judge the size of the shot or infusion I will give myself.

3. Not telling an employee of the car wash that this was an emergency and I needed some candy or a soft drink right away.

4. Not having some emergency glucose or candy in the car.

5. You're now starting to see repetition of some of the same mistakes. Having emergency glucose or candy would have prevented both of these episodes.

6. It would not, however, have prevented the next one.

Christmas 1984

After moving into a spacious family home in the neighborhood of "Turnagain" in west Anchorage, Mary and I began the tradition of having Christmas Eve parties with all our friends who had "Christmas-age" kids. It became a 20-year tradition with Santa Claus, caroling, lots of food and drink, a houseful of excited kids and happy parents.

Christmas Eve 1984 was typical. Our home was festive, fun, and full of friends. Among the big selection of food beautifully presented by Mary in buffet style was a large bowl of shrimp on ice with a smaller bowl of red cocktail sauce in the center.

I remember the shrimp with cocktail sauce because it's one of my favorite buffet foods. As I spent time moving from group to group enjoying the beauty of sharing our anticipation of Santa Claus with friends and family, I would stop periodically at the big bowl of shrimp and pick up two or three large pieces and add a little cocktail sauce. I probably ate a dozen or so pieces of shrimp that evening but very little else.

After everyone had a chance to eat, we all sang Christmas carols waiting for the excitement and chaos of Santa's arrival. As we all sang our traditional "arrival" song, "Here Comes Santa Claus," a big clatter arose on our back deck, I flung open the drapes and there was Santa with a big bag of gifts, one for each of the kids and somehow exactly what they each wanted. The magic of Santa Claus lived for another year in the minds and memories of a few dozen excited little kids.

Everyone helped clean up as they always did, then began leaving to get their kids to bed and prepare for tomorrow morning's evidence of Santa's visit to each home. Mary and I had our same Christmas Eve tradition. After we got each of the kids to bed, we began our typical Christmas Eve activities as Santa's official elves. Mary retrieved all the presents from their hiding places and laid them out under our Christmas tree and around the electric train tracks. I began all the necessary assembly of toys.

Once we were ready for Christmas morning, we headed upstairs to get four or five hours of sleep before the kids would be up and jumping excitedly on our bed around 5 a.m. Just before I went to bed, I realized I hadn't given myself an infusion (shot) of insulin since lunch. Without thinking or measuring, I gave myself 10 units. Eight units would be typical for me for an especially big dinner. I don't know why I gave myself 10 units but it was far too much for having just eaten shrimp and having been very active for the past eight or 10 hours. I knew shrimp or prawns were a low-calorie, high-protein food that required very little insulin to metabolize, but I evidently just wasn't thinking.

Mary and I went to bed feeling very happy, very tired, and very close, and we showed it in all ways. The next thing I remember is three guys in EMT (emergency medical technician or paramedic) uniforms and Mary in her bathrobe standing at the foot of our bed talking. The EMTs had given me a drip of dextrose and water and I was starting to come around. I don't recall what time it was but it must have been around one thirty or two in the morning.

They explained to me that they would have to take me to the emergency room because their policy required it if they had administered any kind of medicine to a patient. Well, the last thing I wanted was to spend Christmas morning in the emergency room so I did everything I could to convince them I was coherent. I started describing what had happened in the evening and to Mary's chagrin exactly what happened when we went to bed. The more detail I covered, the more Mary, who was standing behind the paramedics shook her head "No." I thought maybe she forgot, so the more she shook her head, the more detail I got into. The paramedics were smiling and chuckling and obviously thinking of the great story they'd have to tell the guys back at the station. I was chairman of the Anchorage Assembly at the time and that added value to the story.

As was their policy for the mayor or members of the Assembly, the emergency responders had called Commissioner of Public Safety John Franklin, as soon as the call had come in. Now they called him back to see if they could get his approval to waive the policy requiring them to take me to the hospital. I don't know exactly what the head EMT said to the commissioner but I could hear laughing. He came back into the bedroom, looked at me with a smile and said, "The commissioner asked me to tell you Merry Christmas."

With that, the EMTs packed up and left Mary and me to enjoy one more wonderful Christmas morning with our kids.

Mistakes That Caused This Episode

1. Not measuring my blood sugar before I went to bed

2. Giving myself a thoughtless, uninformed, and inappropriately big infusion of insulin just before going to bed

3. Not knowing at that time that shrimp has practically no impact on elevating blood sugar

Later in this chapter, I spend a lot of time talking about how to avoid *nighttime* low blood sugar problems. It's one of the most commonly occurring and worrisome of low blood sugar events. It is especially worrisome for parents of younger diabetics who so often lie awake worrying about their child's blood sugar.

Yard Sale, Anchorage 1993

In the late spring of 1993, Mary and I decided to take part in the American version of spring cleaning—a spring yard sale. Like many Americans, over the years we had purchased more than we'd discarded. Our attic was full. Our garage was full. My workshop was full. It was time to discard, donate, or sell. I've come to the conclusion that for the first 20 years of our marriage we *accumulated* and for the next 20 years we've *discarded* in one manner or another.

A yard sale it was. Our two sons were away at college but Jen was home to help along with a foreign exchange student from Spain, Victor. It was a moderately sized garage sale that we advertised as starting at nine o'clock on a Saturday morning.

By noon our yard was mostly clear of our once valuable items, which had evolved into space-consuming clutter. While a few people were still showing up, Mary volunteered to go get some hamburgers and drinks. She took orders for Jen, Victor, and me and soon returned with the food. I had asked for a hamburger and a diet soda. When it arrived, I put it on a low brick wall bordering our sidewalk. Then I reached into my pocket, picked out my insulin pump, and gave myself an infusion of insulin. I don't recollect the exact size of the infusion but it was a pretty big hamburger and I would typically give myself a bigger shot for hamburger and a bun than I would for a normal lunch. So I'm guessing I took seven or eight units of fast-acting insulin.

Before I took my first bite, a friend of our boys, Greg Letey, pulled up. Someone had told him we had our lawn tractor for sale. We did and it was still unsold. I put my untouched hamburger back on the low, brick wall in our front yard and walked around to the backyard with him to show him our lawn tractor.

The lawn tractor was one of our biggest items and I recall that we were asking about $400 for it. That was a lot of money for Greg, who was planning on starting a lawn-cutting business that summer to earn money for college. We spent maybe 45 minutes testing it, talking about it, and then doing a little haggling on the price. I recollect that I sold it to him for less than $300.

By the time Greg left, I suddenly realized that my blood sugar was very low and probably going down fast since I had given myself a big shot and had no food going in. Once again the problem of not thinking clearly became an issue. I knew there was a problem but I couldn't logically figure out the best solution. By this time my blood sugar was probably about 40 and going down quickly.

Instead of telling Mary or Jen, who are well informed about diabetes and would know exactly what to do, I tried to solve it myself. I thought about the chocolate and Coke I kept in my nightstand in our upstairs bedroom. With everyone else in the front yard, I began working my way upstairs to the bedroom. By the time I got upstairs, I was confused about where I was. Even though we had lived in that house for 20 years, I couldn't find our bedroom. I kept ending up in the kids' bathroom.

The last thing I remember was trying to find our bedroom by walking slowly toward where I thought it was. I slid my hands against the wall in order to stay as far as I could away from the railing and a 15-foot drop onto the tiles in our foyer below.

Once again I need to rely on family members who were there during this seizure to recall the event as it happened. Mary recalled that our exchange student, Victor, found me as my seizure started. He yelled for Mary. She and Jen ran up the stairs and found me convulsing on the floor. Mary took charge and told Victor, who was a big, strong 18-year-old, to hold me down, and yelled to Jen to call 911. Mary then ran to get a juice or soft drink but recalled, "There was no way I could get it in you while you were convulsing."

Jen remembers thinking, "I was glad Victor was there to hold you and keep you from hurting yourself." An important thing to remember during a low blood sugar seizure is that every muscle is mobilized in the body's attempt to correct the sugar imbalance and is, at the same time, being fueled by a large infusion of adrenaline. Until medical help arrives, it's most important to restrain diabetics and keep them from hurting themselves.

The next thing I remembered was hearing vague voices around me and seeing people in smocks walking around in what seemed to be, through my eyes, a foggy room. My first cognizant recollection was hearing a doctor say, "He's coming around; go ahead and give him three units of insulin." Even in my vaporous state I could feel that my blood sugar was still low and that I didn't need insulin. I managed to tell that to the doctor, who appeared as a hazy figure in front of me. To his credit, he told the nurse to check my blood sugar and sure enough I was still at 50. An additional shot of insulin would have been dangerous. He said to me, "You're right. You're still low." Years later I ran into that doctor at a community event. He came up to me, mentioned that event and thanked me for speaking up.

In rethinking that incident, I realize that even though the paramedics gave me DW50 (in layman's terms, 50 percent sugar and 50 percent water) intravenously, I still had so much insulin going in that although the dextrose raised my blood sugar enough to bring me around, the insulin on board was still lowering it. The doctor didn't know how much insulin I had going in but I did—and he listened to me.

This is one more reminder that diabetes is patient directed. You're in control of your own health. If you can accept that, learn about diabetes, and especially learn from your mistakes, you can have a healthy and long life.

Mistakes That Caused This Episode

1. **The primary cause of this episode was distraction.** I had the food in front of me. I gave myself what I still think was an appropriate infusion of insulin but I let myself get distracted at exactly the time I should have focused on eating. I could easily have avoided the whole episode by simply picking up the hamburger and bringing it to the backyard with me and eating it as I was talking to Greg about the lawn tractor.

2. **The other mistake that contributed was not asking anyone for help.** I have sometimes been able to think clearly enough to ask Mary for help but just as often, I've wandered around trying to solve the problem myself without asking. The fact that very low blood sugar interferes with the ability of a diabetic to ask for help is the very reason that friends or loved ones should ask "Do you need help," if the diabetic seems confused or distracted. It is also equally important that the diabetic not be defensive if someone asks if he or she is okay.

When someone asks me if I'm okay, I've lately picked up the habit of responding and then thanking them for asking. That way people are not discouraged from asking in the future.

A Summary of the Causes of
My Extreme Low Blood Sugar Episodes

Of the nine extreme low blood sugar episodes requiring emergency assistance, the causes break down as follows:

1. *Three* were nighttime lows.

2. *Two* resulted from my not having emergency glucose or sugar handy.

3. *One* was from taking an infusion of insulin without testing first.

4. *One* was from taking a shot for a meal and getting distracted and not eating.

5. *One* resulted from an atypical activity—waterskiing.

6. *One* resulted from a major change in diet to recover from an injury.

AUTHOR'S NOTE:

Five were covered in my first book and the other four in this chapter.

How You Should React to
Low Blood Sugars Based on Urgency

I'm always amazed at how good sweets taste when your blood sugar is low. It's your body telling you that your blood sugar is low and you need something sweet. It's the reason that most diabetics, me included, overreact and eat more sugar than is necessary to counteract low blood sugar episodes.

I'm also continually amazed at how fast certain foods or drinks such as orange juice, apple juice, sugared soft drinks, glucose tablets, or Skittles will enter into your bloodstream. Usually within two to three minutes you'll start feeling the results as your blood sugar goes up.

I've read some books that suggest measuring grams of carbohydrates you take to counteract low blood sugar, then waiting, taking a second measure if needed. In my opinion that's okay for urgency levels one and two listed below but not for urgency level three. Here's the way I categorize my level of emergency action needed in different low blood sugar situations:

Urgency Level One
My blood sugar is low but I have
no insulin going in or on board.

That means no shot or infusion for at least three hours prior to the time I notice the low. This is not extremely serious because my blood sugar is probably not going down very fast. For me this situation is most likely to happen in the morning after my blood sugar may have crept down during the night. I nevertheless don't waste time getting some sugar in (usually Oreos because Skittles taste terrible in the morning). I don't typically need more than one.

Urgency Level Two
My blood sugar is low and I have
both food and insulin going in.

This could be more serious depending on how much food and how much insulin. If I have a substantial amount of food going in and not an exceptionally large dose of insulin, I may wait for 15 minutes and test again to see if my blood sugar is going up or down. If I think I may have given myself more insulin than was necessary for the amount of food I've eaten then it's more serious. In this case I would act with a little bigger dose of some kind of sweets, soft drink or juice and have more handy if necessary.

Urgency Level Three
My blood sugar is low and I have
insulin going in and no food going in.

This is a very serious situation. I may be close to losing the ability to figure out a solution myself and may face impending unconsciousness. In this case either Mary or I will act very fast. Usually mixing Coke with some chocolate syrup, which flattens the carbonation and allows me to drink faster. Speed is important because even after I start drinking it, it's still two or three minutes from getting into my bloodstream, and by that time if I don't stop my blood sugar decline, I could begin a seizure. At that moment I'm not measuring carbs or worrying about overdosing on sugar. My body needs sugar and it's screaming for it. When the sugar starts being absorbed into my blood I usually get back to normal (80–100) and then fly right past that to a high of 200 to 300. Highs are never good, but the consequences of a short-term high are minuscule compared to the consequences of a dangerous low. If I have overdosed on sugar I will—within 15 minutes or so— measure again and add the appropriate infusion of insulin to bring my blood sugar back down to normal.

How You Can Avoid These
Dangerous Low Blood Sugars

Always Test Twice before Going to Sleep—
A Baseline Test and a Direction Test

The most important action you can take as a Type 1 insulin-dependent diabetic is to test your blood sugar twice before you go to sleep. First test about an hour before you go to bed. That's your *baseline test.* Then test right before you lie down. That's your *direction* test.

Two tests will not only tell you what your blood sugar is but which direction you're going. If your *baseline* test is 120 and your *direction* test is between 115 and 125, you're fine and can sleep comfortably, secure in the fact that you're not going to have a dangerous low during the night and will probably not be too high.

If your *baseline* test is 150 and your *direction* test is 200, you know you're going up and you should give yourself enough insulin to bring your blood sugar down 100 points in this example. You now know how to do this using your adjustment factor. In this case I'd give myself two units of insulin because every unit of insulin will bring my blood sugar down 50 points.

If your *baseline* test is 150 and your *direction* test is 100, you need to be concerned about your blood sugar continuing to fall. In this case I would have one Oreo cookie and a small glass of milk or maybe even a half an Oreo with the milk. This decision, though, is more of an art than a science. You want to stop the downward trend of your blood sugar but you don't want to increase it to the point that you're sleeping all night at 150 or even 200.

Keep "Just in Case" Supplies on Your Nightstand

Testing twice is something all Type 1 insulin-dependent diabetics should do but you've also got to be prepared for the possibility that you may make a pilot error. So just in case, you should keep a blood tester, a screw-top bottle of Coke or bottled juice, and a plastic squeeze bottle of Hershey's chocolate syrup or some equivalent sugary juice on a nightstand close to your bed. The reason for the screw top is that I have rarely had a blood sugar low enough to require my drinking a whole Coke. It's usually a sip and a little chocolate. If my blood sugar is in the 70s or 80s, I might have just a sip to assure that it won't get too low during the night. Just to give you an idea of the small size of my adjustments, a bottle of Coke will usually last a couple of months and the squeeze bottle of Hershey's chocolate will last a year or more.

A key reason I keep the Coke and chocolate on my night stand is that if my blood sugar gets too low I can't process my thoughts clearly enough to think about waking up Mary. (If I called her name she would be awake instantly and helping me, but in my confused, low blood sugar state I have rarely, if ever, been able to think clearly enough to awaken her.) The brain needs glucose to function and without it, a confused haze exists. Having a recognizable Coke with its red label and Hershey's chocolate syrup in its brown container on my nightstand seems to remind me in my confused state that I need to drink it right away.

Even though most of my nighttime low blood sugars are mild, I am more likely to experience blood sugar low enough to cause confusion at night than at any other time. If more insulin is going in than is necessary and my blood sugar is slowly going down, I may not wake up until my blood sugar gets down to about 45 mg/dl. By that time I can be confused and unable to focus on what needs to be done. Prior to keeping the emergency sweets in my nightstand, I sometime walked around the house with severe low blood sugar unable to find the kitchen or the refrigerator where I previously kept my emergency Coke. Sometimes after I found the refrigerator, I just stood there with the door open trying to figure out what to do.

Here are two alternatives to consider. First, you certainly can use orange juice or apple juice instead of Coke. They both have about the same amount of sugar and calories as a Coke does. Second, putting chocolate on the nightstand of a young diabetic may be too much of a temptation for the youngster to consume it even when not needed. Glucose tablets are a good alternative for children. But giving the youngster some chocolate is a pretty desirable medicine and that may have some merit.

You May Have to Wake Up at Night More Often Than You'd Like

One of the hardest things to accept is that you may have to wake up a few nights a week to test your blood and adjust. For me this is most often when I've eaten a dinner that's bigger than normal or later than normal. That coincides with a shot that's bigger or later than normal.

If I wake up during the night and am not confident about my blood sugar level, I will typically do a quick test. If it's not between 85 and 110, I may do a slight adjustment: a sip of Coke to raise my blood sugar or a small bolus with my pump to lower it. If, for example, my blood sugar is 120 and I want to bring it down to my typical target of 100, I will give myself .4 units of insulin (it's important to note that is four 10ths of a unit, not four units).

If it's a bigger adjustment, that's a different story. Bigger adjustments in the middle of the night are a little riskier because you're dealing with greater swings (called amplitudes). A blood sugar below 50 or above 250 will usually wake me up…thankfully. I'll wake up and test. The low is pretty easy to solve with a little chocolate and Coke and a quick brushing of my teeth. Then I'm comfortably back asleep in three minutes. A high above 250 or 300 is a bigger problem. I may have to give myself four or five units of insulin and I'm always concerned when I have that much going in at night. In that case I don't quite sleep as deeply and may often wake up again (by habit) in a couple of hours to test again.

All this waking up at night may seem like a big problem. All things considered I'd certainly rather sleep through the night every night. But even though I may often wake up once or twice during the night during a given week, I always seem to be refreshed and feeling good in the morning. Once again, I think it's a matter of attitude. I may not have chosen this road but I sure can choose to walk on the sunny side of it.

Always Have Some Emergency Glucose in Your Pocket or Purse

This would have been a pretty simple solution to at least two of my extreme blood sugar episodes. And it's prevented a few more since

I started always keeping some type of quick sugar handy. My emergency sugar of choice, as I've said before, is the Halloween-size packets of Skittles for my pocket whenever I'm out of the house and a full-size packet for my car, my boat, my fishing tackle box, and my golf bag. I may go months without ever opening a packet but when I do open a packet it's sometimes the only thing between me and a potential seizure.

One of the beautiful little sidelights (please indulge me) of the Skittles is the wonderful interaction this has created between me and my first two grandchildren, Lily and Boden.

Just recently Lily announced to her kindergarten class that her grandpa has diabetes and he has to eat Skittles. It's easy to see how she came to that conclusion because by the time she was two, she knew Grandpa always had Skittles. When she was visiting us I started out by giving her one Skittle after each meal and she was excited about that. Now that she's five, I give her three after each meal. Last summer she figured out the math and declared, "Grandpa, if you give me nine, I'll put them in my purse and promise to eat only three after each meal." She continued, "Grandpa, I always keep my promises." The beautiful thing is that she does keep her promises. She always shows me the three that are left in her little purse for eating after dinner. Boden's following her lead but he's already getting three and he's only three years old.

Never Give Yourself a Shot (Bolus) without Knowing What Your Blood Sugar Is.

Giving myself a shot without knowing what my blood sugar is has caused one *extreme* low blood sugar reaction and a number of other *serious* low blood sugar reactions. In my experience, newly diagnosed diabetics don't do this very often. It starts happening after insulin-dependent diabetics get comfortable and confident that they know where their blood sugar is—or should be.

Years ago I periodically thought my blood sugar was high a few hours after dinner and give myself maybe three units of insulin, enough to bring my blood sugar down by 150 points. Then a half hour later I'd test and find out I was 75 with three units going in. That's a problem, but a small one. I'd just have to eat something else (Oreos and milk in my case). The problem gets bigger, though, if the shot you give yourself is bigger or if you're going to sleep.

Even though you think you know where your blood sugar is and even if you're right 90 percent of the time, that's not good enough. You don't want to put yourself in jeopardy 10 percent of the time because of a judgment that can easily be confirmed or corrected with a 15-second blood sugar test.

Wait Until Your Food Is in Front of You before Giving Yourself a Shot (Bolus)

This is a bit of advice that is not an absolute. Some would argue that it's better to give yourself a shot 20 minutes or so before dinner so the insulin has a chance to start being absorbed by the time you start eating. That's a very defensible argument. It helps match insulin absorption more closely with the blood glucose rise created by eating.

The downside of that strategy is that any delay in eating can be a problem. It's not a big problem if the meal is delayed and you remember you have insulin going in so you can eat something to temporarily hold your blood sugar up. But the real problem is taking the shot and "zoning it out," in other words, forgetting. That's a big problem. You'll remember the shot only when you feel your blood sugar is below 65 or 70. By then your insulin is going into your body full force and since it's before a meal, you'll likely have no food going in to balance it. Then you need to hope you're someplace with sugar nearby or you have Skittles in your pocket. In my opinion, the risk of a serious low blood sugar outweighs the benefit received by giving yourself a shot 20 or so minutes before you eat.

Even my good friend, Al Bramstedt, who has the best blood sugar control of anyone I know (a1c's in the low sixes and even once in a while in the high fives) doesn't give himself a bolus with his pump until he has the food in front of him.

I suggest waiting until the food is in front of you before taking your shot or bolus.

Test frequently during calorie-burning, unpredictable activities

I played in recreational basketball leagues and flag football leagues for about 15 years after I was diagnosed as having Type 1 diabetes and played softball for about 45 years after being diagnosed. In all those competitions, I never had a serious low blood sugar episode.

The reason for my record of all those competitions with no low blood sugars is the predictability and consistency of those sports. I knew how long each of those sports took (about an hour generally) and roughly the energy they took and the amount of blood sugar they would burn. Prior to the availability of self-testing I always ate a candy bar before each of those activities. Since the availability of self-testing, I always test before those activities and can pretty much predict at what blood sugar level I'll be during the games. I always have Skittles, or something similar, with me just in case I'm wrong. It's worked perfectly. No problems with predictable, consistent sports.

The problem I've had with some sports is the unpredictability and the blood sugar surprises that it brings. The two biggest surprises and potential low blood sugar threats for me have been water sports and golf.

To repeat because it's so important, *water sports* tend to bring down blood sugar very fast because they take place in a cold environment which burns energy fast and drops blood sugar very quickly. They can be very dangerous, because a serious low blood sugar reaction in the water presents the threat of drowning. So I am extra cautious about testing my blood sugar and making sure it's at least 180 to 200 when I get into the cold Alaskan water to waterski, wakeboard or wake-surf. Even in warmer climates, if you're in 70-degree water, it's still almost 30 degrees colder than your body temperature and that is going to drive your blood sugar down very fast.

Golf has been the biggest surprise of any sport. A four- to five-hour round of golf burns a tremendous amount of glucose and lowers blood sugar dramatically if the golfer walks a course carrying or pulling a handcart. That wasn't the surprise. But the biggest surprise of all for me was that riding in a power golf cart and playing a five-hour round burns only about 25 percent fewer calories, and therefore lowers my blood sugar about 25 percent less than walking and pulling a handcart. Although golf is not an aerobic sport, it sure is a calorie-burning, blood-sugar-lowering sport.

Atypical and unpredictable activities don't just mean sports, as Mary and I discovered at Disneyland last spring. We had taken our grandchildren, Lily and Boden, to Disneyland for a three-day trip. Lily had fallen and ended up with a scraped knee. I stayed with Boden while Mary took Lily to the first-aid station just off Main Street in the park. While Lily was getting some antiseptic and a bandage, Mary asked the nurse, "What's the most common problem you encounter?" Without any hesitation, she said "Diabetics with low blood sugar." Again, that's an example of an atypical activity that burns a lot of calories and brings blood sugar down faster than expected.

I'm guessing others have had that same problem at any big theme park or carnival. If you or your kids are going to engage in activities that you haven't participated in regularly or activities that burn calories quickly or for a long time, be vigilant with testing before and multiple times during those activities.

If You Get Sick or Are Faced with Recovery from an Injury, Ask Your Doctor What Impact They Will Have on Your Insulin Needs

My only personal experience with an injury that impacted my diet, insulin demand, and blood sugar control was a serious leg burn that I described in my first book. I really haven't been sick much in my life so I don't have much personal experience with the impact that colds or flu might have on your blood sugar. Most of what I've read says your body will need more insulin during those periods, but my only advice is to always ask your attending doctor what he or she thinks about your insulin dosage for blood sugar control during those events.

Chapter 15

Sports, Activities, and Blood Sugar Control for Insulin-Dependent Diabetics

For competitive or active Type 1 diabetics
and thoughts for parents of young,
active Type 1 diabetic children

Testing Before and During Competitive Activities
As you know by now from previous chapters, insulin combined with activity will bring blood sugar down faster than insulin without activity. It is therefore essential that a diabetic using insulin injections or infusions be especially vigilant about testing before and during any prolonged activity.

Testing before a competitive activity is an absolute must. You need to know what your blood sugar (or your child's blood sugar) is and whether or not your blood sugar is going down because of insulin on board. Ideally, you should try to test one hour before the activity starts and then right before it starts. That will give you a trend line, either up or down.

Here's my personal experience summary of appropriate blood sugar levels prior to *competitive* activities:

Above 200 mg/dl this is unnecessarily high unless insulin is on board and no food is on board.

From 150 to 200 mg/dl this is pretty safe as long as the competitor's blood sugar is not trending down prior to the start of the competition.

From 125 to 150 mg/dl this is a risky level for anyone to start a competitive activity. Have a candy bar handy and plan on measuring again in 15 to 20 minutes. If you don't want to measure again in that short time then have at least part of a candy bar before starting. A child can probably get away with eating just one half of a candy bar but anyone over 130 pounds should consider eating a whole candy bar. With the energy that will be burned and the increased blood circulation stimulated, a candy bar under these circumstances will not be a negative influence on long-term diabetic health.

Below 125 the competitor should not start the competition without eating a full candy bar or some other quick-acting, blood-sugar-raising food or drink.

Competitive Activity for Young, Insulin-Dependent Children

There is no reason why a young insulin-dependent child can't take part in any sports he or she chooses. The important action for a parent is to exercise sufficient caution to avoid their child's having a low blood sugar episode during practice or competition but at the same time not communicating a feeling of being overly worried about the child.

If I had an insulin-dependent diabetic child, I would much rather she or he started a competitive activity with blood sugar at 200 mg/dl than at 100. I'm not suggesting 200 as a necessary starting point but somewhere between 150 and 200 will give both you and the child the ability to enjoy the activity and not worry about low blood sugar. As a starting point for competition, 100mg/dl is too low and can be dangerous. I think it's also important to have two candy bars handy at every high-energy competitive activity, one to eat (at least half of a candy bar) prior to the activity if blood sugar is less than 125 and trending down, and one to have in reserve just in case.

If the activity has a halftime, that's also the logical time to test and see how your child's blood sugar is doing. Finally, you should test after the event so you can adjust if it's too high or eat or drink something if it's too low. Testing after the event will also help to better understand that event's impact on your child's blood sugar and give you an understanding of what's best for all similar competitions. The beauty of gaining this understanding is you or your child won't have to worry about blood sugar during the competition.

These recommendations are based on my personal experience competing in sports that involve one to two hours of start-and-stop activity. Tennis, basketball, baseball, hockey, softball, and soccer fit that category. Football is a longer activity with more emotional involvement, so a halftime test is an absolute must and tests at the end of each quarter are desirable. Since I was diagnosed with diabetes as a 20-year-old I have played only in flag football leagues. A flag football game is shorter and less strenuous than a regular football game.

Certainly different people will have different experiences with blood sugar decreases during competitive activities based on weight, aerobic condition, and age. But it's my hope that my experiences and this information will provide at least a starting point for determining how you can best handle your own or your child's blood sugar control during competitive activity.

Testing Before and During Recreational Activities

For long, calorie-burning recreation activities such as jogging, biking, golfing, climbing hills or mountains, walking fast for more than a half hour, or doing any sweat-inducing activity in an athletic club or gym, the guidelines for starting blood sugars can be adjusted down a little from the competition guidelines for two simple reasons: You can test more easily and more often and you can always have some form of glucose on your person and readily available.

Here are my recommendations for appropriate blood sugar levels when starting moderate- to high-energy-burning, *recreational* activities:

Above 170 mg/dl   is unnecessarily high unless you have insulin on board and no food on board.

From 130 to 170   is a safe start for high-energy, high-calorie-burning activities such as those mentioned above. But always have a high-calorie chocolate- or granola-type bar on your person.

From 100 to 130   requires vigilance and attention but is okay as long as you test early and more frequently than if you're starting with a higher blood sugar.

Below 100   too risky to start the activities mentioned above or similar activities. I'd recommend eating half of a candy bar, a Halloween-sized packet of Skittles, or some glucose tablets. The downside, of course, is that you don't want to eat too much because you'll offset some of the weight loss benefit of the activity.

For less strenuous activities such as casual walking, easy biking, gardening, and similar activities starting with blood sugar levels of 100 to 130 is just fine. You should, however check after 15 to 20 minutes just to be sure you're not trending downward.

Type 1 Diabetic Children and Playtime

Because I was 20 years old when I was diagnosed as a Type 1 diabetic, I don't have firsthand experience with childhood diabetes. Although I'm certain that many parents of young children with diabetes have a greater understanding of the impact and appropriate way to deal with diabetes in young children, I will offer the following for consideration.

Since I had diabetes for approximately 15 years before the advent of convenient self-testing, my safest course during activities was to keep my blood sugar high. In retrospect and with the benefit of a much greater understanding of blood sugar levels facilitated by thousands of self-tests, I now realize that always eating a candy bar before competitions without any knowledge of what my starting blood sugars were probably resulted in blood sugars that were frequently in the 200–300 range during competitions. As a result, I almost never had any low blood sugar episodes during competitions.

The pertinent question is, "Did these frequent high blood sugars have an impact on my health?" The answer is—"Probably," but after 50 years it's not clearly evident.

A slight negative result of those high blood sugars from my first 15 years with diabetes showed up, as I said earlier, as slight neuropathy and also as background retinopathy in my eyes when I was 37 in 1981. Now, more than 30 years later with the benefit of self-testing that retinopathy has disappeared, the neuropathy in my feet is diminished and I continue to be very healthy.

My point for parents of young diabetics is this. Although all research points to good control of blood sugars as being important to long-term health, my personal opinion based on my 50 years of experience with diabetes is that higher blood sugars when young kids are playing is not going to result in uncorrectable long-term problems. Their bodies are young and resilient and there is more benefit in letting them (and you) be free from the worry of a low blood sugar episode than any detriment they may experience in the long term from having high blood sugars during playtime.

You still should, of course, work on keeping your child's blood in tighter control during more sedentary times.

A Blood Sugar Strategy for Parents of Young Diabetics

I'm not recommending that young, juvenile diabetics and/or their parents be indifferent to blood sugar control. It's important, and you now have the technology to help measure and control blood sugars. But you need to find a balance between being overly controlling and worried about every high measurement and on the other hand letting your son or daughter be a fun-loving, active child who is comfortable with diabetes.

When a young diabetic is out playing soccer, basketball, football, baseball, or skiing, running, or engaging in any active sport, or just out playing with friends, I wouldn't be worried about him or her playing with a blood sugar of 150 to 200. In my experience, they're much better off starting a physical activity with a blood sugar near 200 than starting an active event with a blood sugar of 100 with both you and the youngster worried about whether they're going to pass out during the game.

During a very active time, blood sugar is very likely to go down. Remember that insulin and exercise or activity both work to lower blood sugar. The two together will lower blood sugar faster than either one individually. The best thing you can do is measure before the activity and after the activity. Then it won't be long before you understand how much a given activity is going to lower his or her blood sugar and therefore at what level you're comfortable starting.

In my opinion, high blood sugars do more harm during sedentary times. The reason for that is that blood sugars often go down more slowly than anticipated because there is little movement to help the insulin lower blood sugar. So when a young diabetic is sedentary or sleeping, blood sugar control should be monitored a little more frequently. I think you'll find that during those times the young person's blood sugar will be higher than you anticipate.

I need to stress that I believe that older diabetics, whether insulin-dependent or not, do not have the same luxury of keeping blood sugars intermittently high. Typically, an older diabetic's circulatory system is not as healthy or resilient as that of younger people, so more vigilance is required to keep blood sugars at normal levels as much as possible.

Three Sports Deserving Special Caution: Water Sports, Golf, and Skiing

Water sports and golf deserve some specific attention because of the surprising and dangerous impact these sports have on blood sugar levels. No sport I've participated in burns calories faster and therefore lowers blood sugar levels faster than water sports. And no sport has surprised me more than golf as a consistent burner of calories and glucose. More than any other sports, these two sports have resulted in more serious and extreme low blood sugars episodes than any other sports.

Snow skiing also deserves some attention because of the potential impact of low temperatures on the burning of calories and glucose as well as the potential for freezing of insulin in tubing that pump users may experience. Personally, skiing has not caused me nearly as many low blood sugar episodes as water sports or golf but cold-weather sports in general pose unique problems.

Water Sports and Blood Sugar

Over the past four years since we built our lake house, I've been taking part in a lot of water sports: waterskiing, wakeboarding and wake surfing. Living in Alaska means the water's not exactly toasty. Whereas we fish "on the lake" about six months of the year, the "in the lake" water sports season here is only about three months: June, July, and August. Most of the time in June and August we use wet suits. In July, when our lake water temperature is usually in the high 60s, we may not use a wet suit or maybe just wear a wet suit top. I once measured 70 degrees in our lake following a series of long, sunny days. I even considered taking a picture of the thermometer in the water, since I considered it as rare as seeing an albino moose, which I would certainly want to photograph as proof of its existence.

As I said before, the problem with water temperature at say, 68 degrees, is that it's still about 30 degrees lower than body temperature. And water tends to drain heat from your body faster than air does. Even with a wet suit on, your body is burning glucose much faster than normally to keep your body warm as well as to fuel the activity you may be taking part in. I've been surprised many times these past three years at how fast my blood sugar drops when I'm both cold and active.

A number of times I've started a water activity like waterskiing, wakeboarding, or wake surfing with my blood sugar safely (I thought) above 150mg/dl and with no insulin going in other than my basal rate of .3 unit per hour. Even though I take my pump off when I'm in the water, my residual basal amount of insulin in still slowly being absorbed. In checking my blood sugar after I climbed back aboard our ski boat after only 20 minutes of these activities, I was often surprised that my blood sugar could drop more than 100 points in that short period.

Dropping from 150 to 50 after just climbing out of the water can be scary on two fronts. First, you're getting close to a blood sugar level that will cause confusion and even a seizure. Second, a seizure in the water would be clearly more dangerous than a seizure on land. Now I don't get in the water for one of these activities unless my blood sugar is at least 200.

The same danger of rapidly dropping blood sugar is present whether you're snorkeling, scuba diving, surfing, or swimming in the relatively chilly Pacific Ocean off the coastlines of California or Hawaii or the Atlantic Ocean even as far south as Florida. Any of the deep-water lakes throughout the United States will lower blood sugars much faster than an equivalent activity on land. Although an extreme low blood sugar reaction on land is somewhat dangerous in itself, the same reaction in water is much more dangerous.

My advice for blood sugar control during water activities is this:

1. Always check your blood sugar before starting.

2. Consider the length of time you will be in the water and whether or not you have insulin on board (*on board* means "going into your body," not on the boat). If you have insulin on board *and* you will be in the water more than 15 minutes, don't start unless your blood sugar is at least 200. If you have no insulin on board and you'll be in the water for less than 10 minutes, then 150 is probably okay.

3. Always have candy bars, a sugared soft drink, or juice handy before starting your water activity.

4. Check your blood sugar after you've completed your water activity. I'm betting you'll be surprised at how much it dropped in a short time and you'll learn what blood sugar level you should start at in the future.

Golf and Blood Sugar

I've been golfing for over 25 years now and it took me many, many rounds of golf to realize how many calories and how much glucose it burns. As you now know, the more calories you burn in an activity, the faster your blood sugar will drop.

I know, I know you're saying, "For goodness sake, how many calories can you burn by riding in a golf cart and taking maybe sixty or seventy swings of a golf club and perhaps twenty-five to thirty-five putts?" The answer is lots of calories and lots of glucose. Golf doesn't do much for your aerobic condition but it sure does burn a lot of calories. I'll tell you later how I've measured the calories burned.

I've had somewhere in the neighborhood of a dozen low blood sugar episodes playing golf—only one caused a seizure and that was about half an hour after I finished. Almost all have happened on the back nine after I've been on the course for two or three hours and when I've been using a golf cart instead of walking. I use carts about 75 percent of my rounds, so that accounts somewhat for the preponderance of low blood sugar episodes while using a cart. But the more likely cause of my more frequent blood sugar problems when I'm riding was my stubborn belief that I couldn't be burning many calories and therefore not burning much glucose using a golf cart for a round of golf. I was wrong.

The most common problem scenario for me would be starting a round of golf with my blood sugar in the 150-to-175 range and no insulin on board other than my base rate. By the "turn" (which means after nine holes) a food shack is usually accessible. I typically tested my blood sugar at that point and found that it had dropped maybe 50 to 75 points to say 100. With my blood sugar at 100 or so, I would typically buy a hot dog, bratwurst, or hamburger plus a Gatorade, vitamin water, or a beer. Though this is not my typical lunch, I would justify it by thinking about all the calories I was burning. The problem was I was burning many more than I ever expected.

For a lunch like that I would normally give myself eight units of insulin. So anticipating at least two hours of activity just ahead, I cut my insulin back to six units. As it turned out so many times, that was still too much insulin for the situation. By the 15th or 16th hole my blood sugar had often dropped to 45 to 55. Blood sugar at that level is not only approaching danger but also has a noticeable impact on hand-eye coordination. I often started shanking or miss-hitting balls. That, of course, is not the real threat. The real threat is a seizure and unconsciousness if the accelerating drop in blood sugar continues. I now cut my insulin dosage by half when I'm playing golf.

Those situations rarely result in an extreme low blood sugar reaction requiring emergency help because I now always have Skittles or candy bars in my bag. I'm also helped by my regular Alaskan golfing buddies, Dave Young, Rick Pollock, and Mike Johnson, who watch for the symptoms and sometimes spot them before I do. Though I do suspect they may hold back from saying anything for a few strokes especially if I'm beating them.

I'd been playing pretty well on our second round of a warm spring day at Hangman Valley Golf Course in Spokane County, Washington in May 2009. In fact, I was two strokes ahead of my closest competitor that round when I miss-hit my drive on the 12th hole. I then shanked my next shot, a fairway wood, and followed up by hitting a really poor 7-iron approach shot. Mike, who is usually the first one to pick up on my low blood sugar, said to Rick Pollock, "Boy, it looks like Mystrom's game is falling apart. He's missed three straight shots. Maybe his blood sugar's low." With some concern, Rick turned to Dave, who was keeping score and riding in a cart with me during the round, and asked, "How does Rick look to you?" Without any hesitation Dave said, "He's two strokes ahead as of the last hole." Although that wasn't the intent of the question, the answer Dave gave compelled Rick to respond by saying, "Well then, let's wait for two more shots before we tell him to check his blood sugar."

They, of course, didn't wait, and asked right away how my blood sugar was. That triggered a test and it was 53 mg/dl, too low. I recollect that I had a triple bogey on that hole. We all took a five-minute break and I ate a couple of handfuls of Skittles—problem solved except I had lost my lead.

A similar low blood sugar reaction happened in March 2012, at another Spokane County golf course. I was playing at MeadowWood Golf Course with a new friend and golfing buddy, Rob Bennedetti. Rob is a doctor at the Rockwood Clinic in Spokane, specializing in internal medicine and nephrology. He and I were playing Meadow-Wood with two of his friends, John Hoye and Blaine Wood. I had been striking the ball well the first 14 holes but on the 15th and 16th my game fell apart. As usual, I didn't immediately think, "Low blood sugar." I just thought " ...a bad couple of holes." But on the tee box of the 17th I checked my blood sugar. It was 55—again too low. Once again low blood sugar manifested itself in the form of loss of hand-eye coordination before I noticed any other symptoms.

How Many Calories Does Golf Burn?

This section is pertinent for any golfers (diabetic or not) who are concerned about their weight.

After my regular blood sugar testing began to convince me that I was burning a lot of calories playing golf even if I rode in a cart, I began to wonder how I could get some more specific idea of how many calories I burned other than "a lot." After some thought I came up with an idea; instead of eating before I started a round of golf and then turning down my insulin pump base rate, I'd start a round without eating, with my blood sugar stable and with my normal base rate programmed in my insulin pump. Under those conditions, my blood sugar would remain stable if I were to spend the next five hours in a normal daily routine. Under those conditions, I started a round of golf, using a golf cart, with my blood sugar as near to 100mg/dl as I could get it. The number of calories I would have to eat during that round would be equal to the number of calories over and above whatever I would burn during my normal daily activity.

By doing this I knew I would have to continually take in calories to keep my blood sugar from dropping dangerously low very quickly. My goal was to end the round with my blood sugar the same as I started with (around 100). The number of calories I had to burn to maintain that blood sugar would tell me how many calories I had burned during that round above what I would normally burn.

I chose Hershey bars without almonds. They are labeled as having 210 calories. I started off by eating one at the first tee box. I continually measured my blood sugar. Every time it dropped back down to about 100 (normal), I'd eat another one. By the time I finished the round, I had eaten four Hershey bars (that's 840 calories *above what I would normally burn during a typical five hours of ordinary activity— sitting and walking*).

I normally burn about 2,400 calories a day—about 100 per hour. Allowing for burning less when I'm asleep, I'm guessing I burn about 120 calories an hour during waking hours. My normal five-hour calorie burn would therefore be about 600 calories.

Add to that the additional 840 calories I burned during that round and the total is 1,440 calories burned while playing 18 holes with a cart. As an additional bit of information, using my pedometer, I've measured my steps taken playing golf using a cart at 7,500 to 7,700 steps.

Golf as a Weight-Loss Activity for Type 2 Diabetics

In general, golf has surprised me in terms of how many calories are burned. I expected a lot of calories to be burned walking a course but I was very surprised at the calories I burned while using a cart. Golf as a calorie-burning activity is important for any Type 2 diabetics or nondiabetic golfers who want to lose weight. The caveat for people in this category is not to overindulge in food after the round. It's very tempting to eat a lot of clubhouse type food such as hamburgers, bratwurst, hot dogs, and fries after your round of golf. You're hungry. You've burned a lot of calories. Why not indulge a little?

The answer is simple (though the execution is harder). Don't waste all the benefit of the calorie-burning activity by taking in more calories than you just burned. Try to moderate your postgolf food. In the examples above, take half of the bun off and don't eat it. Do *not* order fries. Compensate for the smaller amount of food you'll eat by eating more slowly. The same thing goes for whatever you may order: cut the starchy carbs and don't order fries. It's not easy but if you cut out those wasted calories, you'll find that golf will become a weight-losing activity for you.

Precautions to Be Taken by Insulin-Dependent Diabetics Playing Golf

It's important for insulin-dependent diabetics to be aware of these high rates of calorie burning since the rate of calories burned directly affects blood sugar levels and can cause surprisingly fast drops in blood sugar with all its potentially negative impacts.

Here are my suggestions for reasonable precautions while playing golf.

1. Always keep glucose tablets or Skittles in the *same, handy* pocket in your golf bag. "Same and handy" are key words. If your blood sugar drops too much before you catch it, you could become confused and unable to remember in which of the various pockets your emergency provisions are. That can happen. Not often, but it does happen.

2. If you're on a pump, cut your base (basal) rate down by at least half (I cut mine by two thirds). If you're not comfortable

doing this without talking to your doctor, by all means consult her or him.

3. If you're not on a pump you should also reduce the dosage of your injections but so many variables of dosage mixes make it hard to generalize. So talk to your doctor for your specific reductions. Insulin-dependent Type 2 diabetics should also be aware that if you do not reduce your insulin usage for golf or other activities and just eat more to compensate, you're losing any weight loss benefit the activity creates.

4. Always eat something before you start the round and give yourself no more than one half the amount of insulin you would normally give for whatever you eat.

Three years ago, Dave Young and I were getting ready to tee off at Eagle Glen Golf Course in Anchorage. As was our habit, we asked the starter how the pace of play was. "Pretty good," he answered, but then added, "but it's probably going to slow down a little now." "Why's that?" I asked. "Well," he said, "the group just ahead of you guys has a 100-year-old-fellow in the foursome and he's playing a little slow."

Golf is a great game you can play for the rest of your life. Make it a healthy activity too.

Skiing

Skiing deserves a mention here because although it's a cold-weather sport, it burns calories and therefore glucose at a much, much slower rate than cold-water sports.

I do more downhill (alpine) skiing than cross-country (Nordic) skiing but have had no serious or extreme low blood sugar episodes with either sport.

Downhill skiing lends itself to frequent testing because of the frequent breaks riding up a chairlift after most runs. I generally find myself testing my blood after every three or so runs so my control is good and I'll usually catch potential low blood sugars before they get serious.

The other reason I haven't had any serious low blood sugar downhill-skiing is that although certain parts of my body may get cold (face, nose, or maybe hands) my general body core is usually warm so I don't burn as many calories or as much glucose heating my body.

Cross-country skiing is different. An insulin-dependent diabetic needs to make his or her own breaks for testing. It's an intense calorie-burning activity, so cut down insulin input before you start. Eating some sweet or starchy carbs before you start is very important to consider. The activity itself will usually keep your body warm but the colder it is when you start the activity, the more calories you will burn early.

My general advice on both downhill and cross country skiing is that they're plenty safe for diabetics but you need to remain vigilant. Have fun.

Chapter 16

You're the Pilot.
Now You Have the Knowledge.
Take the Controls.

For all diabetics: Type 1, Type 2, Insulin-dependent or not

In the last 24 chapters, you've been subjected to a lot of information. I understand how overwhelming it can be, but by way of encouragement, you don't have to memorize it all. In fact, you don't even have to do everything I recommend in order to be healthy. But you do have to understand your disease and start following as many of my recommendations as you can remember as soon as you can. The reward is you'll start feeling better and more energetic right away and your likelihood of long-term health and enjoyment in your later years will be greatly enhanced.

Learn from Your Doctor but You Are the Pilot

Having a good doctor you can learn from, talk to, and confide in is indispensable. As I've mentioned before, I have the good fortune to have found Dr. Jeanne Bonar, who has helped me for the past 35 years. Dr. Bonar first got me on the pump about 30 years ago. My recollection was that I was the first person to go on the pump in Alaska, but I'm not certain about that. When she first suggested it, I was undecided but she convinced me to try it with a beautifully clear piece of simple logic. "Try it for a month or two and if you don't like it, you can go back to giving yourself shots"—simple, logical, persuasive. I did it and I've been on a pump ever since.

Nowadays Dr. Bonar and I talk more like equals. She brings to the discussion the medical, chemical, and anatomical background that I don't have as well as a lot about the new technology and research. I bring to the discussion a lot of patient perspective information which comes only from living the experience. But no matter how good your doctor is, you are the one who has the control of your own health. Your doctor may teach you how to fly the plane but you're the pilot, you're the one who has to fly it most of the time, because he or she isn't going to be with you all that much.

"My Doctor's in Africa"

Being a well-known diabetic in Alaska results in many people approaching me with questions or observations about their experiences with diabetes. One of the most common observations from diabetics who are unwilling to take control of their disease is that they're having blood sugar control problems and that the next time they see their doctor they're going ask for advice and permission to raise or lower a certain insulin dosage.

Years ago an insulin-dependent diabetic who was the father of one of the boys I coached in baseball told me his blood sugar was consistently high. He was concerned about the fact that his doctor was in Africa and wouldn't be back for a month. He said that his blood sugar was almost always in the 300s and he was feeling a little lethargic and tired but he wasn't going to do anything about it until his doctor got back.

My advice to him was not to let his blood sugar hang around the 300s for another month. I suggested that he start increasing his insulin dosage a couple of units at a time and keep measuring at the same intervals. He'd gradually see his readings get lower. I also suggested another, even better, option: eat smaller portions and fewer starchy carbs. He'd see lower readings by doing that too. Now this was a smart guy. He had a responsible job with the federal government but no way was he going to change anything until he talked to his doctor.

Regrettably, he died seven years later.

Your Doctor Can't Know All the Details of Your Schedule

More recently, a friend of my sons', Tony Mattingly, who had moved to Michigan, gotten married and started a family, lost his job in 2009 (along with about 10 million other Americans). In order to support his family, he moved back to Alaska to try to find a job, while leaving his family in Michigan.

I hadn't seen Tony for maybe 20 years but he knew I was a diabetic and he called me one day and told me his 13-year-old son who was living in Michigan was just diagnosed as a Type 1 diabetic and he asked for some insights. I invited him out for a cup of coffee to give him some background on Type 1 diabetes. He was concerned, interested, and thoughtful. I then invited him to our house the next Saturday and we set up a conference call with his wife in Michigan. We talked for about an hour and she too was very interested and involved.

About a month later, he called back and said his son had started football practice in a youth football league and he was having trouble keeping his blood sugar up. Following their doctor's orders, he was taking a shot before an early dinner, then going to football practice. During practice his son was having repeated low blood sugar problems. According to Tony, "He has to continually try to bring his blood sugar up by drinking colas or eating candy bars until he can't eat anymore." I asked Tony how many units his son was taking before meals and he said, "The doctor has him on 16 units of regular insulin before dinner."

Well, 16 units is a lot of insulin and I'm guessing the doctor probably wasn't aware of football practice after dinner when he suggested that amount. Sixteen units before dinner may have been okay for his usual routine (if there is such a thing as a usual routine for a teenager) but it was far too much insulin on board preceding a two-hour football practice.

I told Tony that the next time he saw his son's doctor to tell him what had been happening but in the meantime, I suggested he cut his son's shot before practice down to about eight units and see how that worked. I told him if I had a son his age with insulin-dependent diabetes, I would much rather have him start practicing at 200 mg/dl than at 100. When a young boy like that is out playing football it's much more important to focus on avoiding lows than worry about highs. Let him play football without worrying about a low reaction. Let him go out there and be a boy and have fun. I don't know if Tony and his wife followed my advice or not but I'm guessing that they did because of their interest and willingness to learn. I'll also bet that their son is enjoying football more and is more likely to continue with more athletic activities and be healthier because of it.

Now certainly there are people reading this book that are saying, "The author's not a doctor, how can he advise someone to change insulin dosage?" Well, every day all over America, diabetics are talking with one another, giving advice, asking for advice, telling about experiences, and just generally learning from each other. The more they communicate the better they become at knowing what to accept, what to try, and what to reject. It's an informal "sharing of diabetic living experiences" going on all over America and probably the world, and it's making us all healthier.

You can't do it without a good doctor or medical professional to get you started and help you along but he or she can only teach you how to "fly the plane." She can't anticipate the universe of situations you will face. Your doctor may be the instructor but you're the pilot. You've got to make the decisions that will enable you to live a long, healthy life with diabetes.

Remember this. Probably more than any other disease, diabetes is patient directed. You're in control of your own health. If you can accept that responsibly, learn about diabetes, learn from my mistakes, and every bit as important, learn from your own mistakes, you will live a long, healthy, active, and I hope a "wonderful life with diabetes."

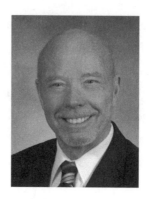

About the Author

Rick Mystrom was diagnosed with Type 1 diabetes in 1964 while attending the University of Colorado at Boulder. Instead of denying the reality that was diabetes, he chose to shape that reality into living a healthy, bold, and active life with diabetes and added a promise to never complain about having diabetes.

In 1972 Rick and his young family moved to Alaska, where he started and operated two successful businesses. Just nine years after moving to Alaska, he was named Alaska's Small Business Person of the Year and one of America's top three small businessmen.

He served two terms on the Anchorage Assembly and was elected to two terms as mayor of Anchorage. He was elected chairman of the Alaska Conference of Mayors and was twice selected as Alaska's Elected Official of the Year. He also served as chairman of America's Olympic Bid Committee for the 1992 and 1994 Olympic Winter Games.

Now at 70 years of age, and a diabetic for 50 years, Rick is a paragon of good health. A recent stress test categorized him as equivalent to an "active 42-year-old." He credits his good health to good eating habits, an active lifestyle, and an understanding of foods. For nearly

30 years, he has tested his blood 5 to 10 times a day and has a unique understanding of which foods contribute to good health and which detract from good health.

For the past three years, Rick has meticulously measured, organized and graphed—in a way never before done—the impact that different foods and combination of foods have on blood sugar and weight gain or loss.

That information in this book means lower blood sugar and weight loss for Type 2 diabetics and better blood sugar control for Type 1 diabetics. And for the two thirds of all American adults who are anywhere between slightly overweight and obese, this book is your answer to a longer, healthier, more enjoyable life.

Presentations Worldwide

Rick has given presentations nationwide on diabetes and worldwide on the Olympics. The reactions to his presentations are always enthusiastic.

Here are comments from a keynote presentation he made at the Rockwood Clinic's Diabetes Day in Spokane, Washington. Because of the response to his presentations there, he has been asked to make two keynote presentations in recent years to accommodate the expected crowds.

Audience Comments

"Rick Mystrom was a terrific speaker.
He had great clarity in his presentation.
It was personal, practical, and enjoyable."

"Number seven speaker, (Mystrom), was wonderful."

"I Enjoyed Rick Mystrom. He was very encouraging and upbeat."

"Please repeat Rick Mystrom—*Living with Diabetes.*
We missed it and were told it was excellent."

"Really liked the mayor from Alaska, Rick Mystrom"

"Rick Mystrom was the best." "Excellent." "Awesome"

"I like surprises. Rick Mystrom's, *Living with Diabetes,*
was a delightful surprise."

"When you have speakers like Rick, who have so much
to share, please allow them more time."

If you would like Rick Mystrom to speak at any diabetes related or weight related group, you can contact him at Rick@rickmystrom. com or by phone at 907-440-7425. You can also communicate with him via his web site at Rickmystrom.com.

Recommended Reading

Bernstein, R. K. . *Dr. Bernstein's DIABETES SOLUTION: The complete guide to normal blood sugars*. New York: Little, Brown and Co. 2011 February

Davis, L. *Is this any way to lose weight?* Reader's Digest, 80-93. February, 2011.

Davis, Dr. William. *Wheat Belly*, New York: RODALE, 2011.

Taubes, G. *Why we get fat*. New York: Anchor Books. 2011.

Weil, Dr. Andrew. *Dr. Andrew Weil's Guide to Living Longer & Better*. OneSource Content Marketing LLC. 2013.